Bring Out Your Dead

THE GREAT PLAGUE OF YELLOW FEVER
IN PHILADELPHIA IN 1793

By

J. H. POWELL

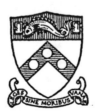

Philadelphia
UNIVERSITY OF PENNSYLVANIA PRESS
1949

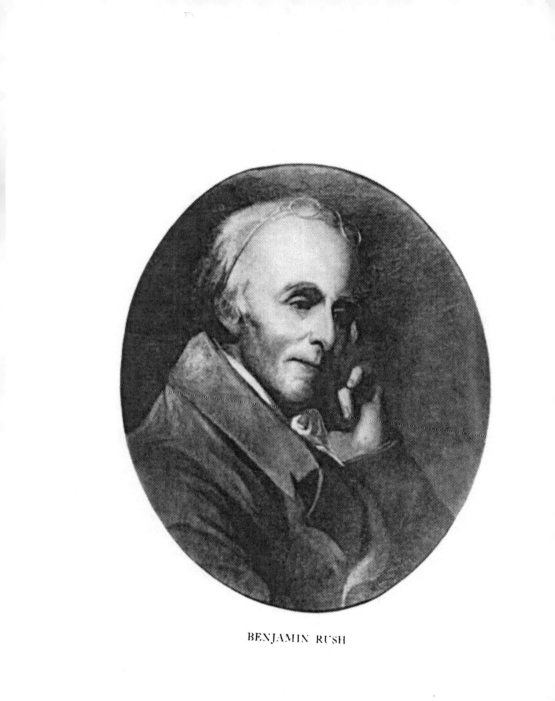

BENJAMIN RUSH

Preface

*Perhaps by writing no man can express
What people suffer'd in this great distress!*
—SAMUEL STEARNS

Do not read this book before eating, or in the midst of a sleepless night. For it is a revolting book, filled with disgusting details of a loathsome disease. And unfortunately, all the details are true.

As true, that is, as men's knowledge of the truth ever is. So great was the tragedy, so astounding the scenes of suffering, that one after another of those who lived through the plague wrote down what they saw. They are responsible for all the facts recorded here; and if they sometimes saw things that could not happen, told stories beyond belief, that is because they were men, not cameras. The historian can never construct a record of events. All he can do is construct a record of records.

The Yellow Fever in Philadelphia in 1793 is one of the great tragic episodes in the human history of this land. It was the most appalling collective disaster that had ever overtaken an American city. For a century afterwards, the fearful disease remained an annual threat for people in many states and many towns to dread, and every year they remembered the great Philadelphia plague as the worst, the most frightening, the very classic of plagues. The yellow fever is gone now, and the record no longer helps us in preventive medicine. But the human values of those hundred days of horror remain, with all the cowardice and courage, the cynicism and faith, the knowledge and the vanity that people have.

This is the story of a foul and fantastic pestilence, striking

v

without warning in all classes of society. It is the story of people sick in body and heart, astonished and fearful, paralyzed by the mysterious obscenity about them. Men, said Epictetus, are tormented with the opinions they have of things, not by the things themselves. Yet this is torment, none the less, and leaves scars deeper, uglier, angrier than a saber wound.

Philadelphia was a low, level town, hottest and dampest of all the American seacoast, hotter even than Charleston, Savannah, or the West India cities, people said. Wharves jutted out into the river and cut off the current; high tide deposited rotting stuff on the banks and in the mud. Below the city were swamps, marshes, pools in clay pits, stagnant water. Most of the streets were unpaved. There was no water system, and only one sewer, under the serpentine of Dock Street. Elsewhere holes were dug, as at Market and Fourth streets, to receive water from the gutters. These "sinks" exhaled a noxious effluvia, for dead animals and all kinds of nauseous matters were hurled into them to putrify. All the wells were shallow; citizens continually pronounced them polluted.

In 1793, Philadelphia had about 55,000 inhabitants. Ordinarily, some 2,500 were born every year, and every year around 1,400 died. Many of the citizens were German-speaking, many French; 2,500 were Negroes. The middle-aged had lived through the American Revolution; even boys in their teens could remember when the treaty of peace had been signed ten years before.

The city was America's national capital—temporarily, for Washington on the Potomac was being built; but until 1800 the government was by the Residence Act decreed to remain in Philadelphia. The greatest figures in public affairs gathered here: this plague was an incident in George Washington's life, and John Adams', Thomas Jefferson's and Alexander Hamilton's. It precipitated a quaint constitutional crisis; it also affected politics. John Adams, who liked to make things seem bigger than they were, wrote that only the Yellow Fever of '93 saved the United States from a revolution of government.

But the plague was the whole people's problem, not the giants' only. Though the great men weave in and out of the story, the heroes of this book are the little people of Philadelphia, men history usually forgets—the mayor Matthew Clarkson, the tavern keeper Israel Israel, the merchant Caleb Lownes, the music master Andrew Adgate, an umbrella maker, a cooper, a one-legged blacksmith, the warden of the jail.

And Stephen Girard, hero of Bush Hill, a man so extraordinarily gifted in courage and charity that Philadelphians never afterwards understood him, but stood in uneasy awe, suspicious that so much goodness should live in a Frenchman and a man of trade.

And two Negroes, former slaves, whom white men had insulted in a house of God, but who now were the first to show that fear could be conquered by the spirit of Christian love.

And the doctors—those wonderfully learned, disputatious, enquiring, credulous eighteenth-century doctors, who stood between medieval and modern medicine, proud of traditions and systems millenniums old, enchanted by experiences as new as the great new world. For all their abundant observations and good sense, the doctors had but to name a thing to make it real, had but to find a theory to cure the ills from which men died.

Today, because of the heroism of Walter Reed and his volunteers, we know that the yellow fever is not contagious, cannot be defeated by fumigation or isolation, has nothing to do with thunder, lightning, or the new moon. Reed discovered that it is carried from one person to another by a female mosquito, known as *Aëdes aegypti*. *Aegypti* is an especially fierce biter in the early afternoon. If she bites a yellow fever victim in the first three or four days of his fever, the germs of the disease pass from the patient's blood into *aegypti's* stomach. During the next twelve days, they migrate from her stomach into her salivary glands, from which she discharges them into the next person she bites. After she is infected, *aegypti* can inject the disease into a different human being every three days, which is as often as she feeds, and can go on doing so as long as she lives, which is roughly until frost.

She causes a ferocious sickness, usually fatal. It begins with chills and pains in the head, back, and limbs; temperature rises rapidly to a great height, bowels are costive, urine scanty and albuminous. This lasts a few days. Then the fever declines, and sometimes the patient appears to have recovered. But a remission follows, after which temperature rises again, the victim turns yellow, throws up a stale blood, black in color; hemorrhages occur in the intestinal mucous membrane. Last comes a typhoid state, marked by stupor and hebetude, dry brown tongue, rapid feeble pulse, incontinent faeces and urine, rapid wasting. From the external symptoms the disease takes its common names, the Yellow Fever, or the Black Vomit. The patient's appearance is ghastly, the stink of the sickroom overpowering.

Now, because we know the carrier, we have erased the yellow fever from temperate zones. Scarcely a doctor practicing in the United States today has ever seen a case, or would know what to do if he saw one. But in 1793 neither doctors nor anyone else knew the significance of the mosquito. Varro, an ancient Roman, had warned farmers not to build their houses on swampy ground, "because certain animals, invisible to the eye, breed there, and, borne by the air, reach inside the body by way of the mouth and nose and cause diseases which are difficult to get rid of." But eighteenth-century scientists had abandoned such notions of tiny monsters in the air, sinister and invisible. Instead, they realized that the air itself was composed of molecular fluids and solids, and somehow, they felt, these became infected.

They were good observers, these doctors. They described the disease accurately, with faithful attention to detail. And they all mentioned the large number of mosquitoes, even though they comprehended no connection between the two. They stood, confounded with the fever, as we stand today with polio or cancer. They cannot be condemned. We should regard them, as their leader Dr. Redman regarded his predecessors: "Yea, tho' we may with some reason, from the enlightenment of medical science since, smile at their mode of theorizing . . . let us rather pay all due respect to their memory and give them all the credit we can. . . ."

To one, we can give an abundance of credit. This book, though it deals with a whole city in plague, is necessarily a book about Philadelphia's most amazing citizen, Dr. Benjamin Rush. "The American Sydenham," people called Rush. He was the greatest among great teachers, when Philadelphia was the medical center of the whole country. He was a father of modern psychiatry, leader of a new school of practice, founder of an American tradition. He remains to this day the most imponderable single figure in the history of medicine in the new world. No one since Rush has gained such mastery over the whole profession.

The plague of '93 was Dr. Rush's greatest moment. His accounts of the fever, in lectures and books, spread his fame everywhere books were read. And his private letters in his heroic labors are among the most appealing literary achievements in the language.

Indeed, my difficulty has been to place Rush in a proper perspective, for it is all too easy to feel, as he unquestionably felt, that others were misled where he was shown a great light, others indifferent where he was first in devotion. Dr. Rush's radiant charm is seductive. I find I sometimes forget, in the spell of his presence, that he had no common sense. But sense that is common is also dull. And dull, Dr. Rush never was.

Mathew Carey helps with the perspective—Carey, the Irish-born publisher, historian of the plague. Some said his successive tracts describing it saved him from bankruptcy. And the writings of all the others—the diarists, the doctors, the citizens—help, too. Some could even write as though Dr. Rush had never lived. It was a gross error on their part. The French doctors—the wonderful Devèze, Dr. David Nassy, the elusive M. Robert who suddenly turned up in Philadelphia from the Philippine

Islands—these shrewd, cautious physicians of an alien culture unquestionably saved lives. Rush unquestionably spent them. But a plague is not a matter of science, a calculus of life and death. It is a matter of the soul. Rush felt this. He knew one more thing than the scientists knew (for in the true sense, he was not a scientist)—he knew that truth is no physical thing, but an element in the moral structure of life, unprovable, unseen.

Historians are dependent on their sources. Had I more time and ability, I should have made this book a novel, for there are so many things the sources do not tell. There are heroisms unrecorded, great moments of beauty and courage that have left no trace, unknowable human experiences that would teach wisdom and understanding. I wish Matthew Clarkson had told his story, and Caleb Lownes, and Peter Helm. I feel sure Dr. Hodge must have been a man of sturdy heart and fine abilities. And what must Stephen Girard have seen!

But history is always full of gaps. And looking back over the sources, I am a little surprised that so much is really here in the record, so many individual people somehow emerging a little more than just a name, a little more than life-size, for a moment at least, in the long stream of things that men have thought, and done, and said, and felt.

Acknowledgments

THE staffs of the Free Library and the Library Company of Philadelphia have given invaluable help in the preparation of this book, as have the librarians and staffs of the College of Physicians, the Historical Society of Pennsylvania, the American Philosophical Society, the Connecticut Historical Society, the American Catholic Historical Society, and several other institutions. Henry Adams was most courteous, helpful, and generous. Many friends and many people who heard me talk on this plague furnished special information. I owe particular thanks to Margaret J. Duxbury for patient help with the manuscript.

Catherine Drinker Bowen read the manuscript through in its various stages, devoting many days to patient criticism. Lois Given, Charles Lee, and David Appel did likewise, and Lyman H. Butterfield read the sections dealing with Dr. Rush. Richard Harrison Shryock studied the whole book and made numerous suggestions. Venia T. Phillips gave me the benefit of her knowledge of entomology. Harold A. Spilman, M.D., Martha A. Bell, R.N., and Carl Bucher, M.D., were most helpful in medical details. Erwin Clarkson Garrett, Joseph Sickler, Mr. and Mrs. Joseph Carson, Nicholas B. Wainwright, Charles F. Jenkins, Mabel Zahn, J. Bennett Nolan, and many others supplied numerous suggestions and out-of-the-way material.

To these, and to others who have been interested and encouraging, I extend sincere thanks.

Contents

List of Illustrations

Pestilence

Written During the Prevalence of a Yellow Fever

Hot, dry winds forever blowing,
Dead men to the grave-yards going:
    Constant hearses,
    Funeral verses;
Oh! what plagues—there is no knowing!

Priests retreating from their pulpits!—
Some in hot, and some in cold fits
    In bad temper,
    Off they scamper,
Leaving us—unhappy culprits!

Doctors raving and disputing,
Death's pale army still recruiting—
    What a pother
    One with t'other!
Some a-writing, some a-shooting.

Nature's poisons here collected,
Water, earth, and air infected—
    O, what pity,
    Such a City,
Was in such a place erected!

—PHILIP FRENEAU
Philadelphia, 1793

"*A Merry, Sinful Summer*"

*. . . when the heats come on soon, and continue
throughout autumn, not moderated by winds, or
rains, the season proves sickly, distempers appear
early, and are dangerous.*—SIR JOHN PRINGLE

SPRING came early in 1793. The winter had been mild, with no
snow and only moderate frosts. Streams had not frozen. In
January it was so warm that Philadelphians could lie on their
backs on the bare ground watching the balloon ascension of
the famous M. Blanchard from the Prison Yard.

By the first of April, fruit trees were in blossom, and birds
returned two weeks ahead of time. May was uncommonly wet.
Day after day a dismal, driving rain, cold and relentless, poured
from the northeast. People kept their fires burning far later
than they had for years. Swollen streams overflowed their banks,
creating new marshes and swamps in the lowlands and the
city's alleys.

June turned suddenly warm, and the summer proved the
hottest, driest, dustiest even the oldest inhabitants could remember. Rivers sank to rivulets and creeks dried up, leaving
their new marshes behind them as small stagnant pools. Drainage in the streets and primitive sewer system ceased almost
entirely. The entrails of fish, the rotting carcasses of dead animals, the refuse of the city piled up on the Delaware's bank and
in the city's markets. A foul stench was wafted gently westward
up the High Street.

The dry spell became a drought, the drought a disaster. Pas-
tures dried up, grains shriveled. Where a stream two or three
feet deep had been, men could walk dry-shod in the hot sun

1

amid the buzzing of mosquitoes. Water in the city's wells sank below pump level. Had fire begun it would have raged unchecked. Apprehensively, Philadelphians recalled destruction wrought by an arsonist during the drought two years before. What criminal design had done then, mere chance could outdo now.

But fire was not the only danger. Discomforts of the summer brought other ills to mind. As they endured the torment of "an amazing number of flies and other insects," Philadelphians thought with dread of the familiar "autumnal disease," that annual affliction of late summer and early fall, inescapable scourge of the city's year. "Summer complaint" old wives called it, or autumnal fever or heat sickness or the fall ague. It could be serious, especially when other diseases were about, and there certainly were other diseases this year. The strange weather had brought all sorts of sickness: mumps in the winter, influenza and scarlet fever in the summer, other fevers in July as the drought began to have its weary way. Hippocrates had observed, as any medical student at the University knew, that "when the winter has been too mild, or too cold, when the spring or summer, and the following autumn have been dry, we must fear cruel diseases." Everyone noted the uncommonly numerous mosquitoes, which all authorities pronounced "a certain sign" of unwholesome atmosphere.

Some foul thing was loose in the air of Philadelphia that year, indeed in the air of all America. People counted the signs, month after month. Dr. Rittenhouse had seen a comet in the constellation of Cepheus. Oysters all up and down the coast were watery and inedible. Nature unaccountably burst into savage life, as up in Kensington in July when lightning struck out of a blue sky and split a noble old oak into eleven pieces, or in Ipswich where a sudden tempest of rain and hail one summer's afternoon had cut down fields of grain and flax, stripped the fruit off trees, broken thousands of window glasses, while less than three miles all around the day had remained hot, dry, and calm.

In the great heat farmers dropped in the fields, because, country folk said, there was no wind and the sweat dried slowly on their bodies. Country folk could tell the auguries of other signs—large numbers of wild pigeons had always meant unhealthy air, and never had the city markets seen so many wild pigeons as were sold in the stalls in 1793. Strange diseases were attacking animals, diseases like the "yellow water" afflicting horses in New Jersey and cows in Virginia.

People told these things to each other, and read them in their newspapers. Elsewhere there was sickness, particularly, it seemed, in river towns where drought dried up the streams. Vermont suffered influenza and a putrid fever, Harrisburg and Middletown in Pennsylvania had many unexplained deaths, Dover in Delaware had "an extremely fatal" bilious disorder, Virginians had the flux—there in a few weeks five hundred inhabitants of five counties fell "the unhappy victims of this depopulating disorder."

Sweltering and dusty in the August heat, Philadelphians endured the summer ills and waited for the fall. The red brick houses shimmered in the haze. Along the waterfront where docks and jetties trapped the river's dirty water the stink was unendurable. Steams and vapors rose from the marshes to the south, and in the Northern Liberties, where city gentry had their summer homes, the parched earth turned to ashes.

Yet even in August heat the streets were thronged with people. Philadelphia was America's national city, her political capital, her greatest port of trade, and seat of much of her learning. It would take more than a summer's heat to halt the busy routines of such a city. People went to stores and markets, churches, alehouses, clubs. They gathered in groups on the street corners, they picnicked in the public squares or dined down at Gray's Ferry Gardens on the banks of the lovely Schuylkill. Federalists held dignified processions for President Washington and neutrality, Republicans in rowdy crowds sang the *Ça ira,* danced the *Carmagnole,* feted Citizen Genêt, and demanded war with England. Summer heat brought no end to politics.

No end to excitements, either, for Philadelphia had some unexpected guests that hot, dry summer. In July one ship, then another, then whole fleets of ships came in from the West Indies, discharging from their crowded holds great hordes of refugees, white, black, mixed, from the French island of Santo Domingo. Gaunt, hungry, sickly, they poured into the city, bringing news of a great revolution in the sugar islands, of a horrible carnage and slaughter, of the destruction of towns and the ruin of merchant houses.

They told of three years' warfare, how the slaves rebelled, and how the great port of Cap François had flamed against the sky. They told of a pestilential fever which had ravaged the islands—Grenada, Dominica, Hispaniola, Jamaica, even Barbados, Antigua, and all the Leewards. They told of an agonizing voyage on fever-ridden ships, a voyage of people who had lost every worldly possession and watched the burning of their homes, of people exposed to the hot sun by day, crowded by night into the closest quarters, of people unclothed, with no food or provisions, of people tragically delivered from a ghastly terror. "Would to God I had the courage to take my life and escape from the horror of such a cruel recollection," one of them wrote.

For weeks the ships kept coming, and for weeks Philadelphians witnessed the pitiable spectacle of husband seeking wife, parents children, families hoping to unite, strangers in an alien land begging news of each other. "If the misfortunes of Santo Domingo should have obliged either of the partners of the house of l'Enfant & Chevalier, of Cap François, to take refuge in this country," read a notice in Brown's *Federal Gazette*, "or Mr. Godefroy Beutier, inhabitant of the district of Rozeaux, quartier of Jeremie, or the daughter of Mr. Grehault de la Motte, of Nantes; they may hear of something interesting, by applying to B. & E. Carnes, No. 71, Second-street." Trade with the islands stopped, and with other ports as well, because of the failure of credits and destruction of merchant-house records at Cap François. Refugees were starving and penniless. They continually besought Philadelphians for money, clothes, food, and news.

For weeks they kept coming. By the end of July the number passed a thousand, by the end of August it exceeded two thousand in the city and suburbs—two thousand high and low born, of all skills, trades, and professions, all indigent, all in need of immediate help. Other cities had taken them in, too. More than a thousand had gone to Baltimore, and there in one hour $11,000 had been subscribed for their relief. Newport, Charlestown, New York were all raising funds. Philadelphians were determined not to be outdone. There were already many Frenchmen in the city: refugees from revolution in Old France and citizens who had come over in the days of our own war for independence. They could help. Stephen Girard, Peter Duponceau, and Peter LeMaigre had already organized a *Société Française de Bienfaisance de Philadelphie.* Let them provide relief, find homes for the Santo Domingans near the waterfront among their own people, find jobs, clothes, and food. Meanwhile native Philadelphians, proud of their century-old tradition of benevolence, would raise money. A committee was formed, subscriptions taken, more than $15,000 collected. John Bill Ricketts, "the celebrated equestrian," gave a benefit performance, so did the theatre company. Distribution of funds began, by people who could speak French. Soon much of Philadelphia, long bilingual with the German population, learned a third language as well.

Few cities of fifty-five thousand could ingest and absorb two thousand strangers without a serious dislocation of social life. But Philadelphia, ever since the first French refugees had come, and then the whole bureaucracy of the federal government, had been a fluid sort of place. The Santo Domingans were just one more housing problem.

They were not easy to place politically, however. They said they were Republicans, and had favored the French Revolution, but to Philadelphians they were a handful of whites who had protested about the rights of man while trying to keep half a million blacks in slavery. The French Revolution was the central issue of American politics. Neighbor split with neighbor over the neutrality question. And refugees of all opinions were living evidence to Philadelphians of all opinions, of the good or evil they saw in disasters abroad.

The Santo Domingans were not at once accepted in the city's life. Fine doctors, great merchants, experienced lawyers were among them, but Philadelphians, uncertain of their strange political allegiances, asked no advice, showed no curiosity.

Of sympathy, however, they gave abundantly. Even pro-British Federalists were shocked by the stories of the voyage: how English privateers had preyed upon the overfreighted ships, boarding and searching, making prizes of vessels owned by Frenchmen, seizing refugees' property on American ships, taking prisoners. British captains had not been too scrupulous. They had treated American vessels with appalling highhandedness. The Philadelphia brig *Mary* had been stopped out of Cap François by a privateer whose crew confiscated the property of a hundred and fifty refugees on board, tore up the cabin floors in search of hidden goods, took off five Negro girls and all the wine they could find. A few days later the *Mary* was overhauled by another Britisher, whose crew stole everything remaining and scuttled the brig's water butts. Victims of such savagery deserved every kindness a city could give, political questions notwithstanding. The Santo Domingans found their way eased.

Newspapers began to publish items in French; dancing academies, fireworks manufactories, fencing salons, hairdressing parlors, and many another enterprise of French culture sprang up. The refugees were being assimilated.

They found their new home in many things puzzling, in many delightful, in all things interesting. The regular, geometrical plan of the streets, the orderly substantial brick houses, the many churches of many sects, the cemeteries right in the midst of town, the thriving commerce and expanding industry, the windows that opened up and down like a guillotine, the 662 tri-formed street lamps that burned every year 8,606 gallons of oil, the handsome State House, the broad and airy High Street, the narrow, airless side streets—these and innumerable other sights of Philadelphia made the first city of America a sharp contrast to Cap François, the Môle, or Port-au-Prince of the plantations, or the cities of Old France.

Philadelphia was a new and fresh experience for the refugees; so were they for Philadelphia. Their *insouciance,* their cleverness in occupations, their street games and songs, their ready adjustment, their avid participation in the cock fighting, rope dancing, gambling, taverns, theatres, and alehouses of Philadelphia contributed to give the city, in spite of the heat and drought, what the Reverend J. Henry C. Helmuth termed "a merry, sinful summer."

It was a strange year.

Infection in Water Street

There was something however, in the state of the atmosphere in the city, or in the constitution of the inhabitants, peculiarly favorable to the operation of the contagion. . . . —DR. WILLIAM CURRIE

ON Monday, August 19, Dr. Benjamin Rush emerged from his house in Walnut Street, just above Third. The day was cloudy, a little cooler than usual lately, with a gentle northerly breeze. Walnut Street, its line of red fronts broken by the open ground of the Friends' Almshouse across the way, had a settled and prosperous look, as indeed it should, for settled and prosperous people lived there. Philadelphia could boast some handsomer streets, with more elegant homes, but it had a great many not so handsome parts, too. Respectable and convenient, only a couple of squares from the High and about the same distance from the waterfront, Walnut at Third was an ideal location for a doctor's establishment.

Rush turned down Walnut Street, passed Judge Peters' fine place on the corner, and began purposefully to stride toward the river. Gray, forty-seven, fastidiously clothed, slender and erect, he was a familiar figure among Philadelphians in 1793. He never walked too rapidly, for he had a chronic cough and a weakness of the lungs, which he had long treated by bleeding himself occasionally, watching his diet strictly, and accommodating his dress, as he urged everyone to do, to the highly changeable climate of the city.

The practices the Doctor urged everyone to adopt, hygienic,

8

social, political, moral, were legion, for Benjamin Rush was an inveterate espouser of causes. But this day his mind was on other things, and as he trudged down the hill across the meandering curve of Dock Street and turned north up Second, he gave his attention to some puzzling medical problems.

Yesterday he had lost a patient, Mary Shewell, twenty-five-year-old wife of the prosperous Baptist merchant, Shallows Shewell. Yesterday also his friend Peter Aston had died of a strangely violent disease that looked just like Mrs. Shewell's. Aston had been a patient of Dr. Benjamin Say, who had asked Rush to consult with him. The doctors had found the good merchant in a wretched state, sitting on the side of his bed, "perfectly sensible, but without a pulse, with cold clammy hands, and his face a yellowish color." Rush prescribed "the strongest cordials," but Aston died in a few hours.

Nor had Mrs. Shewell and Peter Aston been the first. Fully two weeks earlier Dr. Hugh Hodge, who lived in Water Street above Vine, had called in Rush to see his little daughter. Hodge was a stubborn, crusty man, but he had been a Revolutionary army surgeon and was well established in the medical profession. Rush found the child feverish and bilious, her skin yellow; she died in two days. Thomas Bradford, the printer, had sent for him to see his wife, who showed the same violent symptoms of a fever—bloodshot eyes, headache, melancholia, parched throat, nausea. Happily, she recovered. Rush had given her a purge of calomel, and bled her twice. She was up and around now, though her eyes and face were still yellow in color. John Weyman, a patient of Dr. Young, had been delirious and nauseated when Rush saw him. The moment he died his body turned gray as lead and "issued a cadaverous smell."

To lose a patient was always a catastrophe for Dr. Rush. Death was a moral and professional enemy; his complicated mind was forever suggesting reproaches and omissions after a defeat. As he proceeded up Second Street, the breeze in his face, in front of the City Tavern, past the Bank of Pennsylvania in Lodge Alley where he used to live, and the Dispensary in John

Guest's house at the corner of Chestnut Street, other recent experiences were fresh in his memory.

From Mrs. Bradford's he had gone to see a young boy named McNair in great distress, feverish, with eruptions on his skin, nauseated, throwing up a black, grainy vomit, and given to nosebleeds. He bled and purged, but the boy died. Two Palmer brothers on Chestnut Street had been seized one after the other, but they had responded to treatment. So had Mrs. Thomas Leaming; but in all cases the vicious, violent symptoms and morbid yellow color had been noted in the Doctor's daybook.

Rush crossed over Chestnut Street and kept on up toward the High. August heat was an unsavory thing. It seemed to embalm every stale and pungent odor. The breeze carried the foul smells of the great market in the High down to Rush's sensitive nostrils. Rotting sheep's heads and the entrails of yesterday's cattle were certainly not the most pleasing odors in the city. The street was filled with people, most of them Santo Domingans jabbering in French. Dr. Rush, glancing down toward the river, could see the masts and spars of the vessels that had brought them making an intricate lattice against the sky.

Past the Friends' Meeting House, across High Street through the market, on up Second by Christ Church and the Baptist Meeting, Rush made his thoughtful way. He turned right on Arch Street (some people still called it Mulberry), went east a square and more across Front Street. Halfway down the hill he turned left into the narrow alley that was Water Street— "the narrowest, yet one of the most populous in the city," a contemporary wrote; "the street is only thirty feet wide, and but a little above the surface of the tide: the houses are high, and the greater part of them have no yards, particularly those situated on the West or bank side; an inconvenience which tends much to render the street more nauseous. It is much confined, ill-aired, and, in every respect, is a disagreeable street." Up the dirty, dusty way Rush plodded, past the rear of Stephen

Girard's home, until he reached No. 77. Here he stopped. It was the house of Peter LeMaigre, successful French importer who had lived some years in the city, and was now busily engaged in finding money, food, clothing, and jobs for the Santo Domingo refugees.

It was not a part of the city Dr. Rush frequented much, nor did he particularly know M. LeMaigre. But Dr. Hodge and Dr. Foulke had been treating the Frenchman's lady, and they had asked Rush to join them for consultation. Hodge's house was just a few doors up the alley, and the back windows of Foulke's Front Street home looked down over Water Street and the wharves. John Foulke, former student of Rush, was now a Fellow of the College, and sat on the hospital board. He also lectured in anatomy. The three men represented knowledgeable Philadelphia medicine. They met on a grim business.

Engaging, active, pious Catherine LeMaigre, thirty-three years old, was desperately ill. She complained of a great heat burning in her stomach, she vomited constantly a black bile, she gasped and sighed. The doctors conferred, but they could do nothing. Cathy LeMaigre was dying most horribly, in the same manner Peter Aston and Mrs. Shewell and the others had died. It was a formidable thought.

As the three sobered men left her chamber, they paused for deliberation. Rush gravely remarked that he had seen "an unusual number of bilious fevers, accompanied with symptoms of uncommon malignity" lately. He suspected, he said, "that all was not right in our city."

Dr. Hodge, his own little daughter so recently dead, agreed, remarking that this savage fever had carried off no less than five persons within sight of LeMaigre's door. Clearly something was happening in Water Street. Dr. Foulke spoke of cases of his own, and called attention to the stale, pungent smell in the air. This, he observed, had a perfectly obvious origin. The sloop *Amelia* from Santo Domingo, crowded with refugees, had carried a cargo of coffee, which rotted on the voyage. The damaged coffee had been dumped on Ball's Wharf a block away on July 24 and had putrified there, "to the great annoyance of the whole neighborhood."

This news brought Rush up short, and he seized upon it avidly. All his patients—Dr. Hodge's child, the McNair and Palmer boys, Mrs. Bradford, Mrs. Leaming, John Weyman, Peter Aston, Cathy LeMaigre—had been in this neighborhood. Their infections could obviously be traced to the noxious effluvia of the rotting coffee. So could the illness of a blacksmith's apprentice who worked at Race and Water streets, and of Elizabeth Hill, wife of a fisherman infected by "only sailing near the pestilential wharf." Once the discrete cases were thus shown to be related, the disease could have a name. Rush remembered his student days, and the plague of thirty years before. With the coffee as the unifying principle, his cases presented the picture of an epidemic.

There in Cathy LeMaigre's parlor he had his revelation. He did not hesitate to pronounce the disease the *bilious remitting yellow fever*. This was Monday, the nineteenth of August. In less than a week, Philadelphia was a shambles.

II

The words "yellow fever," as soon as Rush pronounced them, spread an uneasy fear throughout the town. From house to house went the news that a malignant, mortal disease was abroad. Some refused to believe it. Rush advised his friends to leave the city, but doctors who had seen no cases scoffed at the advice and declared the fever nothing but a severe form of the autumnal disease. To trouble the public mind by crying "epidemic" was no light thing. Rush was ridiculed and detested, but he insisted on his diagnosis, and during the next few days went busily about urging preparations against the coming disaster.

Disaster it would be indeed, if the yellow fever were really here. A city could resist invasion or repress riot—these were human things. But no people could combat a scourge which

moved unseen, uncomprehended, unyielding through the sense-
less air.

For a whole week after that Monday when Rush emerged
from Cathy LeMaigre's, men and women discussed his grim
words. To some it was no surprise. The air had been polluted
all year, the drought had raged all summer. Would it be so
strange if Dr. Rush were right?

Not strange, perhaps, but what a ghastly tragedy! Philadelphians knew the yellow fever. They feared no disease more.
Happily, for thirty years they had not seen it, but many times
in the long ago frightful pestilence had come and wrought a
fearful havoc. Yellow fever was part of Philadelphia's history.
Back in William Penn's time when the city was new, people had
been mysteriously seized with the hideous disease. Old Isaac
Norris had written about it. He called it "quite the Barbados
distemper—they void and vomit blood." And every decade for
seventy years the visitation had returned, each time more dreadful than the last.

No one had ever known what it was, or what had caused it.
Some said it came from the filth of the city, from the marshes
and swamps, and the open sewer of Dock Creek, that "large
and offensive canal" which wandered through the most populous parts of town. But most Philadelphians hated to think of
disease arising from their own "salutiferous" air. They insisted
it came from abroad. First they called it the Barbados fever.
Then for a while, when they noticed how sick many of the
German immigrants were, they called it the Palatine fever.
Finally, Pennsylvania troops went to fight in the West Indies
in the 1740's and came back with the disease. This seemed to
make sure it belonged to the West Indies. Quarantine acts were
passed to keep it out; a port physician was appointed. Fisher's
Island in the Delaware below the city was purchased and a pest-
house built on it; thenceforth the place was officially known as
Province or State Island, though people familiarly called it
Mud Island.

But quarantine failed to stop the yellow fever. Observing

this, some Philadelphians decided the disease was not imported
at all. They pointed again to local conditions befouling the air;
they demanded sanitation, for they said the putrid miasmas
arising in the city impregnated and infected the solids of the
aether. These, not bodily contagion, transmitted the disease.
This became a major controversy in medical theory. Contagionists would prevent fever by quarantining incoming vessels from
sickly regions; climatists would purify the city and society itself
by sanitary measures.

Both sides had their arguments and their innings. One story
was still being told to prove West India origin: how the elder
Samuel Powel (father of Dr. Rush's friend) had sent a lad as
supercargo to Barbados, where he died of yellow fever. His
clothing and dunnage were sent back to Philadelphia; his
mother, father, and aunt came to get the chest. In the presence
of Mr. Powel, a friend, the three relatives, a cooper, and a clerk
in the counting house the chest was opened. So vile a stench
poured forth that everyone in the room sickened with the fever.
Mr. Powel and several others died.

But different stories were told, too: how when Dock Creek
was paved over and made a street, people near-by used fewer
ounces of bark every fall than they had pounds before; how old
Dr. Bond had contended again and again, through five visitations of pestilence, that it was local in origin, had some relationship to stagnant water, that cleanliness would prevent it. Dr.
Bond told everyone to bathe in the "sulphurous chalybeate
waters" of Philadelphia springs. Waters "properly impregnated
with the chalybeate principles" would strengthen digestion,
counteract the summer sun, dilute the thick, putrid bile, and
destroy "the effect of a hot, moist and putrid atmosphere."

It was an old controversy. Everyone knew it, everyone had
opinions on it. And many who heard Rush's warnings could
remember the plague of 1762, when hundreds had died of the
silent, sudden malady that struck without cause or warning in
all ranks of the people. It was a frightful plague, a famous
plague, a dismal one, and it had solved nothing. Contagionists

had traced it to a West India ship coming to Sugar House Wharf below South Street, from which three men were landed, or to a vessel from Havana tied up above South Street from which a sick sailor was stealthily transported after dark to the house of one Leadbutter, where he died and was secretly buried. Leadbutter, his whole family, many others in the neighborhood, and soon people all over the city succumbed.

If not the ships, what had caused it? No one knew. But as Rush issued his statements, people recalled that it had come suddenly, after fifteen years of freedom from yellow fever. Perhaps now the freedom of thirty years would bring no greater immunity.

And of course everyone could see the Santo Domingans. They were all about. Dr. Rush was a climatist, as old Bond had been. But he could be wrong about the origin, even while he was right about the existence of the disorder. Common fevers—the jail fever, camp fevers, the eruptive military fevers, the autumnal remittent—all these could arise locally; but for a pestilence as terrible as yellow fever some new element was needed. The refugees were this new element. They were sickly, they told of fever in the islands. Why should they not have brought the Barbados distemper, the Siamese fever, the Burmese, the West India, the spotted yellow fever with them? Surely here was an argument to support Rush's contention.

III

Some physicians knew quite well that Rush was right, for his diagnosis solved their problems. If only they had been able to talk to him sooner, tragedies might have been averted. Bright and witty young Isaac Cathrall, for example, back in the first week in August had begun to notice an unusual concentration of sickness and deaths around Richard Denny's lodginghouse in North Water Street. Denny's was a favorite resort of sailors and new arrivals, to which many of the Santo Domingans and men of Genêt's privateer *Sans Culottes* and her prize *Flora* out of Marseilles had found their way. It was not a whorehouse, as some have said, but a simple Water Street rooming place of the cheaper kind, situated between the red frame houses of the block where Dr. Hodge lived and the nest of dirty yellow dwellings up toward Callowhill Street.

To Denny's Dr. Cathrall's professional duties took him on August 3 to examine Mrs. Richard Parkinson, an Irish woman who since June had lived there with her husband and two daughters. She was suffering with a strangely violent malignant fever, for which Cathrall treated her. That night an Englishman in the same house fell suddenly into a stupor and died. Dr. Physick came at the request of the Guardians of the Poor to do a post-mortem, but found nothing except "some derangement in the colon and vessica fellis" and the vessels of the brain "uncommonly distended and turgid with blood."

Two French sailors had taken a room at Denny's. One of them was stricken with fever, and though attended by a French physician living near-by, he died. On the seventh, after four days' illness, Cathrall's patient Mrs. Parkinson died. Next, Mr. and Mrs. Denny themselves sickened and expired within a few hours of each other. Finally, the other French lad died. At the house adjacent to Denny's ordinary the same severe and vicious seizures killed two persons.

Now all of these cases had occurred before Peter Aston's death, or Mrs. Shewell's, or Catherine LeMaigre's, but they were among humble people and foreign sailors, and the doctors who saw them were either French and Santo Domingan, or young Americans of no prominence who practiced among the poor of Water Street because they were just making their start. Cathrall, not yet thirty, had returned from his Edinburgh, London, and Paris studies only a few weeks before, and Philip Syng Physick, just twenty-five, had been home less than a year. Physick, whose father had found him an office in Arch Street near Third, had begun practice with two shillings sixpence in his pocket. He knew the Priestman family, and had established himself by a sort of medical insurance plan whereby Priestman and some other heads of families gave him $20 a year to act as their physician. This and his work for the Guardians was supporting him by the end of the summer.

These young men could have furnished Rush with important facts. But not until the great men saw patients of their own, not until the disease had struck at the respectable orders of society, not, in short, until the fever was several weeks old, could the great men be convinced, and the plague properly begin. If only Rush had stumbled into Cathrall back on August 5 when he went up Water Street to see Dr. Hodge's child!

Or, if only Dr. Foulke had not made such an effect with his news about that coffee. For there had actually been fevers and deaths far removed from the stink of the rotting filth on Ball's Wharf. Up in Kensington, where Dr. Say practiced, a carpenter had died, and several Danish sailors had been seized with rigors, shooting pains, violent temperatures, the black vomit, and hemorrhages. Down in Chester the master of the xebec *Sans Culottes* had died of a violent fever, and a number of other seamen had been put ashore ill before that vessel and her prize *Flora* had come up to the wharf near Denny's ordinary. Plenty of doctors believed from these signs that whatever was happening to the city came from abroad—from the West Indies—and had nothing to do with the Philadelphia air or its pollution by stench and offal.

Rush was confident, however, from his "discovery" of the coffee, that the air was befouled, and a fever of local origin abroad. Doubting nothing, he went to see Mayor Clarkson and Governor Thomas Mifflin, he conferred with other doctors, he did what he could. On Wednesday, August 21, he wrote his wife (who was summering in Princeton with her family) that the fever had not yet spread beyond the reach of the coffee's putrid exhalation. By the end of the week, however, it was breaking out elsewhere.

"You can recollect how much the loss of a single patient in a month used to affect me," Rush wrote. "Judge then how I must feel, in hearing every morning of the death of three or four!"

IV

Indeed, deaths suddenly increased, as though to name the disease were to cause it. On any average August day Philadelphia would have three to five burials, but two days after Rush's discovery the totals began rising, to twelve, thirteen, even, on Saturday, August 24, to seventeen. The church bells tolled endlessly. On that Saturday Frederick Starman, merchant, "died after a short illness." In Water Street Thomas Miller, merchant, and his only son succumbed, as did five other persons in the same region and four in Kensington in the space of a few hours. "The fever has assumed a most alarming appearance," Rush wrote his wife on Sunday, August 25. "It not only mocks in most instances the power of medicine, but it has spread thro' several parts of the city remote from the spot where it originated."

Mayor Clarkson, in his office in the new City Hall, listened to Rush with judicious attention. He was a judicious man. Of course, if there was a mortal disorder, everything possible must be done, but exactly what steps could be taken? Mayor Clarkson was no alarmist. He was a sober, substantial, tough-minded man of business, just how substantial and tough-minded the whole of America was soon to learn.

Matthew Clarkson at sixty was everything all Philadelphians wished to be. Rich, amiable, learned, pious, important in the world's affairs, happy in his home, and useful in good works, Clarkson was the perfection of a middle-class ideal. Behind him lay a lifetime of achievement. Like so many who have served Philadelphia well, like Stephen Girard and Benjamin Franklin, he was not a native of the city. He was of the New York aristocracy, descended from a provincial governor on his father's side, from great patroon families on his mother's. But he was orphaned in his youth and had to make his own way in the world. He started as a clerk in one of the Philadelphia merchant houses engaged in western trade. As a young man, complete with ruffled shirt, silk stockings, and kid gloves, he had ridden to Pittsburgh on his company's business, commandeered a river boat, gone down the Ohio and Mississippi clear to Kaskaskia where he traded with the French *habitants,* studied the Indians, and actually composed a vocabulary of the Osage language. Back in Philadelphia he practiced surveying and engineering, gained some reputation in astronomy and mathematics, turned to insurance, and as trustee of the Mutual Company (the Green Tree) rose to be one of the principal underwriters of the city.

By 1793 he had amassed a considerable fortune, but he had nine children to provide for, and with nine children no man can be idle. Yet he found leisure for both private and public employments outside of business. The intelligentsia of Philadelphia knew him as councilor and treasurer of the American Philosophical Society, and as friend and executor of the estate of the learned Pierre du Simitière. The public at large had first known him before the Revolution, when he was notary public and for a while judge of Common Pleas. During the war he served as auditor of army accounts, then as marshal in Admiralty and receiver of prize goods. Patriotically, he contributed great sums to support Washington's army. He had helped found the Bank of Pennsylvania, once he was elected to Congress (but never took his seat), in 1790 he became alderman, in 1792 the rest of the aldermen had chosen him mayor.

Little could happen to upset Matthew Clarkson. He had all the self-confidence that high birth, high adventure, high-church Episcopalianism give a man, all the poise that comes from much learning, hard-won success, and a houseful of children. His qualities were universally recognized. Jeremy Belknap found "something singularly good in him, a benignity that beamed in his countenance," though it must have beamed rather crookedly, for Matthew Clarkson's countenance was marred by a strabismus or heterophoria, because of which his two dark eyes peered steadily in different directions.

Dr. Rush knew that the Mayor had little actual power. He was merely a presiding officer; real authority belonged to various committees of the council. Both on regular and special occasions, committees were appointed. Committees were the way of democracy. The Mayor could not act without them, and even with them he was subject to influence, if not control, by the Governor.

Yet Clarkson as mayor was the symbol of municipal authority, the embodiment of corporate life. To him Rush naturally turned. He told the Mayor that the strange disease was carried by putrid miasmata in the air, that it originated locally from the filth and corruption about the city, that the thing to do was remove the filth. Accordingly, on Thursday morning, three days after Rush left LeMaigre's, Clarkson announced in the papers that there was "great reason to apprehend that a dangerous, infectious disorder" prevailed. He commanded the scavengers immediately to clean the streets and gutters in every part of town, and "as fast as filth is laid together" immediately to haul it away—where, his honor did not say. He proposed that Water Street be cleaned first; next all the alleys thence into Front Street, then the more airy streets.

"I expect," the Mayor observed, "that the inhabitants will have the satisfaction of seeing this business going on, this afternoon or tomorrow morning; any delay on your part will reasonably be considered as an improper attention to a very essential duty."

Actually, neither the funds existed nor the will to act with the expedition Clarkson enjoined, but some steps were taken, among them the publication in the newspapers on Saturday, August 24, of the old law requiring householders to clean the walks and gutters about their premises and place their rubbish in a heap in the street every Monday and Thursday so the scavengers could collect it next morning.

The spectacle of garbage, paper, and filth blowing about the narrow, dusty streets waiting for the scavengers was an abomination to Philadelphians. A writer for Brown's paper, aroused by the fever, described it over the signature "A Hint":

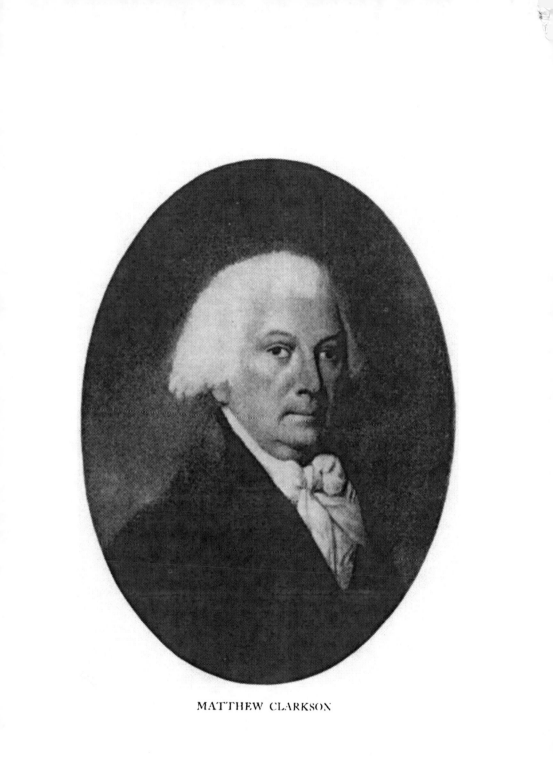

MATTHEW CLARKSON

The practice is to put the offals consisting of bones, with some flesh on them, the entrails of poultry, and many other corruptive matters in a barrel, in the yard, and in some cases in cellars, where they putrify, and are very offensive, and must infect the air with a nauseous destructive quality, and I think less injury would probably follow, from throwing them at once into the street, where the dogs would devour the meat, and the cows the vegetables, than keep them collected in a mass, until in a state of corruption, of which we are witnesses; when the dirt-casks are brought out to be emptied, the smell of which, is scarcely supportable. It would be better, we should pay an additional tax, to have the Scavengers call at our houses three times a week, than thus be sowing the seeds of death, in our own borders.

Of course the Mayor realized that cleaning up the city might not stop the fever, for there were those other doctors who said fevers of this kind were imported, and not, as Rush held, of local origin. An authentic opinion on this matter would help. Clarkson asked that the College of Physicians convene and give its advice, so a meeting of that body was fixed for Sunday, August 25.

Meanwhile Governor Mifflin, with the legislature's assemblage only a week off, found himself as much concerned as Mayor Clarkson over Rush's news. He instructed Nathaniel Falconer, Health Officer of the Port, to ascertain the facts concerning the existence of an infectious disorder, where it prevailed, when it was introduced, what caused it, and what should be done; he asked the Port Physician, Dr. James Hutchinson, to find out if a contagious disease existed, and if so what was its nature; he wrote to Mayor Clarkson asking him to coöperate with Falconer and Hutchinson in this enquiry.

Dr. Hutchinson was a Fellow of the College, calm and sensible, an able man much admired. On receipt of the Governor's letter he went about taking the opinions of various doctors. He was an impressive figure, "as large as Goliath of Gath," usually to be found on the opposite side of any question from Dr. Rush, and certainly not ready on this occasion to accept Rush's opinions without careful examination. Rush found Hutchinson (so he said) denying the existence of any kind of pestilence, and consequently on Saturday, August 24, composed a most careful letter to the Port Doctor, asserting that there really was a fever, highly malignant, caused by the putrid coffee on Ball's Arch Street Wharf; that it had spread into Second Street and up to Kensington, but, he remarked with a sudden access of caution, "whether propagated by contagion, or by the original exhalation, I cannot tell." He omitted his confident diagnosis of yellow fever, saying only that the disease had all the symptoms of "a mild remittent, and a typhus gravior"; he added that he had not seen a fever of such malignity since 1762.

Hutchinson went on gathering opinions Friday and Saturday; Rush went on spreading his news; more and more doctors were called to see more and more cases. It was obvious that the College would have a great deal to discuss on Sunday. It was also obvious that the doctors were not going to agree.

v

Fifty-five thousand people learn things slowly, and learn them with different degrees of conviction. Rush, ubiquitous as he seemed after that Monday when he left Catherine LeMaigre's, could not be everywhere. The first thing most people knew of their danger they learned from the papers. On Friday, August 23, two small notices were published.

One paragraph recommended as preventives against "the present raging sickness" diffusing tobacco smoke and sprinkling vinegar throughout the house, placing tarred rope in a room or carrying it in the pocket, and hanging a camphor bag about the neck. A second suggested that the fire companies "cause their engines to be exercised daily" in flushing the streets, which would relieve the sickness and at the same time keep the engines in working order.

Many people began lighting bonfires in front of their houses or at the corners of the streets to purify the air, a practice attended with serious dangers in the dry August heat. On Saturday a writer who signed himself "A. B." argued in the *Federal*

Gazette against fires, proving from records of plagues in London and Charleston that such a remedy never arrested infectious disorders. The same writer on Monday, August 26, urged that church bells be silenced, for their constant tolling at funerals had a depressing effect upon the sick.

"A. B.," whoever he was, kept busy writing the next week, and contributed to *Dunlap's American Daily Advertiser* on the twenty-ninth one of the most remarkable paragraphs of the plague year, of which, of course, no one was to see the full significance for many generations:

As the late rains will produce a great increase of mosquitoes in the city, distressing to the sick, and troublesome to those who are well, I imagine it will be agreeable to the citizens to know that the increase of those poisonous insects may be diminished by a very simple and cheap mode, which accident discovered. Whoever will take the trouble to examine their rain-water tubs, will find millions of the mosquitoes fishing (?) about the water with great agility, in a state not quite prepared to emerge and fly off: take up a wine glass full of the water, and it will exhibit them very distinctly. Into this glass pour half a teaspoon full, or less, of any common oil, which will quickly diffuse over the surface, and by excluding the air, will destroy the whole brood. Some will survive two or three days but most of them sink to the bottom, or adhere to the oil on the surface within twenty-four hours. A gill of oil poured into a common rain-water cask, will be sufficient: large cisterns may require more, and where the water is drawn out by a pump or by a cock, the oil will remain undisturbed, and last for a considerable time.

Personal safety concerned everybody. "W. F." recommended camphor in the nostrils and mouth, and in a linen bag "put to the pit of the stomach," or, if preferred, the famous "Vinegar of the Four Thieves," the complicated receipe for which he got from Poulson's new *Town and Country Almanac*:

Take of Rue, Wormwood and Lavender, of each one handful; put these altogether with à gallon of the best vinegar into a stone pan, covered over with paste, and let them stand within the warmth of a fire, to infuse for eight days—then strain them off, and to every quart bottle put three quarters of an ounce of camphor. Let the camphor be dissolved before it is put into bottles. Rub the temples and loins with this preparation before going out in a morning, wash the mouth, and snuff up some of it into the nostrils, and carry a piece of sponge that has been dipped in it, in order to smell to pretty often.

This was the recipe said to have been discovered by four young men during the plague at Marseilles in 1720, and used by them with such success that they were able to move safely among the sick and dead and rob them while pretending to be nurses.

People searched out their copies of Defoe's description of London's great plague of 1665 and conned them avidly for remedies. Rush had a first edition, given him by a friend. He underlined, made marginal notes, and added observations in the back leaves. Less professional readers noted with encouragement that a London gravedigger and pallbearer had avoided infection by the simple expedient of chewing garlic and rue and smoking tobacco, while his wife, a nurse, had suffused herself with vinegar and likewise escaped illness.

Among the nostrums proposed was the practice recommended anonymously in Bache's newspaper by Dr. Benjamin Duffield, of strewing fresh earth in a room to a depth of two inches and changing it every day. This Duffield described as "a most comfortable and sure antidote" which the cautious person could supplement by frequent warm baths and "the Asiatic remedy of myrrh and black pepper."

A boy, learning that tar was a sure preventive, tied a tarred rope twice around his neck at night and buttoned his collar over it. He awoke strangling, just in time to tear it off. "He may with justice be said," Mathew Carey observed, "to have nearly choaked himself to save his life."

Gradually the notices increased, and during the next week Philadelphians found the fever occupying more and more of their attention; but the life processes of a great city could not easily or quickly be disturbed. The inertia of commerce kept people going to and from their business houses in the stifling heat, worried perhaps, but needed, doing the thousands of jobs that preserved the subdivided economy of urban society. Socially, Philadelphia was a highly complicated structure, a struc-

ture which had just been described by the Latin master James
Hardie, A.M., in his *Philadelphia Directory and Register,*
offered for sale in July by Thomas Dobson at his shop in Second
Street for five-eighths of a dollar.

In one-line, alphabetical entries, Hardie listed the busy deni-
zens of a thriving community, engaged in their numberless
occupations. In his lists, individual personalities were sub-
merged; fortuitously, great and small alike were reduced to a
strange commercial anonymity, for the city, not its leaders, was
Hardie's theme. Samuel Pemberton brewer and James Pemberton gentleman stood in his book side by side, as did Benjamin Rush M.D. and Benjamin Rush rigger. One entry read,
with no prevision, "Girard Stephen, grocer, 43, No. Front St."

There were graziers and butchers, carpenters, painters, nailers
and cordwainers, widows galore; coopers and hatters, merchants and saddlers, skin dressers, joiners, tailors and carters,
whitesmiths and blacksmiths, mariners, chandlers, brushmakers,
weavers, grinders and cutters; stablers, wool combers, plas-
terers, gentlemen; druggists, curriers, captains, and milliners;
hucksters, tobacconists, aldermen, turners; brokers and soap
boilers, farmers and potters. One inhabitant was listed simply as
"invalid," others as "blackball makers"; there were "mustard
and chocolate manufacturers," "saddlers, bridle-cutters and
harness makers"; and early parking-lot attendants near the
markets and theatres were described as "keepers of horses and
chairs."

The Minister Plenipotentiary from Great Britain Hardie
listed between two widows, as he did Secretary Alexander
Hamilton; Governor Thomas Mifflin was accompanied by a
sugar refiner and a War Office clerk; Chief Justice John Jay
was not listed, nor was Vice-President Adams, but Secretary
of State Jefferson, who lived down at Gray's Ferry, followed
just after a boardinghouse owner. Succeeding "Wartman Adam
merchant" and before "Wassem Christopher labourer" came the
name "Washington George, *President of the United States,*
190, High St."

The people, great and little, who made up the city of Philadelphia differed scarcely at all from people great and little
everywhere. They reacted slowly to advice in the papers, and
to the news of Rush's warnings. A plague is compounded not
of disease alone, but of people's reaction to disease, how they
recognize the pestilence, how they fear it or flee from it or fight
it, how they are unnerved or gather resolution to conquer it.
Rush's diagnosis of yellow fever did not make a plague; it only
started that bewilderment and wonder which would soon turn
to horror in the general public mind.

Newspapers and doctors were not the only advertisers of the
fever. Preachers were talking of their experiences. The Reverend J. Henry C. Helmuth of the Lutheran Congregation had
an uncommon number of funerals. On August 19 he was called
to a man whose breathing was short and who died on the
twentieth; another in the same family died the next day. The
Santo Domingan relief committeemen were finding people desperately ill. Clerks failed to show up at their countinghouses,
printers at their shops; along the waterfront stevedores, sailors,
haulers, and chandlers were telling of sickness in their families.

Even more effective than conversation in advertising the
plague, however, were the smells everyone could smell, the illness
everyone could see. Irresistible arguments supported Rush's
fears. Those markets—there were three of them—were large and
busy. The one in the High Street extended for three long blocks,
through all of which the rotting refuse of a week lay foul and
putrid. Front, Second, Third, and Fourth streets from Arch to
Chestnut would be chained off on market days (Wednesdays
and Saturdays) to accommodate the throngs in the great
market; the Second Street stalls were opened Tuesdays and
Fridays. Cleaning up afterwards was a casual process.

The drought meant low water in the river, and the banks
were lined with a slimy mud shingle where decaying carcasses
of animals and fish had drifted; and as for that coffee, the facts
as they emerged were clear enough. The sloop *Amelia,* William
Williamson master, had actually landed in mid-July with the

captain and five hands sick. Rotting coffee had truly been dumped on Joseph Ball's Wharf above Arch Street, and put up for auction on July 30 "on account of the concerned." No buyers had come forward, and now after another month, Prothonotary Charles Biddle was ordering the coffee sold and removed. It stank terribly. Anyone without medical prejudices could easily imagine it the cause of infectious exhalations.

By the end of this first week, the fever was grimly advertising itself. Scenes which reminded Rush of his histories of true plagues began to confront him as he moved through the streets. In homes through the settled part of town, persons of all ages were being stricken. Lassitude, glazed eyes, chills, fevers, headaches, nausea, retching, and nosebleeds would suddenly attack people in the best of health. These symptoms, more violent than any the doctors had ever observed, would be followed by a yellow tinge in the eyeballs, puking, fearful straining of the stomach, the black vomit, hiccoughs, depression, "deep and distressed sighing, comatose delirium," stupor, purplish discoloration of the whole body, finally death.

It was quick and desperately severe. In one case it killed in twelve hours, though it usually reached its crisis in four days. Curiously, it was accompanied by angry little eruptions on the skin, inflamed and sore—petechiae, the doctors called them. They itched. Rush noted these eruptions, which, he observed, "resembled moscheto bites." They were red and circumscribed. "They appeared chiefly on the arms, but they sometimes extended to the breast. Like the yellow color of the skin, they appeared and disappeared two or three times in the course of the disease." Such petechiae were, he added, in most cases "harbingers of death."

By Saturday, August 24, grief and fear had visited home after home; the strange, insidious disease had claimed victim after victim. What could the common man do? Through *Dunlap's American Daily Advertiser* that Saturday, "Philanthropos" addressed the physicians, praying that since the mortal disease seemed to be infectious, and might become epidemic, would they not join together and recommend measures for Everyman to adopt by which he could avoid the disease? Perhaps by exchanging ideas they could even arrive at a cure.

The doctors, at least those who belonged to the College, needed no such urging. They were already amply prepared for their meeting on the morrow.

Fever, Domestic and Foreign

AUGUST 25–26

I hope I shall do well. I endeavour to have no will of my own. I enjoy good health and uncommon tranquility of mind. While I depend upon divine protection, and feel that at present I live, move, and have my being in a more especial manner in God alone, I do not neglect to use every precaution that experience has discovered, to prevent taking the infection.—BENJAMIN RUSH, August 25

ON Saturday, August 24, rain fell; and on Sunday the twenty-fifth a northeast storm struck with savage force. That Sunday, as dust turned to mud in the city streets and winds blew with great strength, citizens began to leave town. By carts, wagons, coaches, chairs, by horse or on foot, overland or across the rivers, a huge throng of Philadelphians, those who had somewhere to go, streamed out to the country, shutting up their houses entirely or leaving servants in residence, sometimes forgetting to leave them funds.

Charles Biddle, en route back to Philadelphia from a vacation at Yellow Springs, met the hordes moving out and heard their melancholy tales of the fever, including the news of his friend Peter Aston's death. He sent his children to his brother-in-law's country seat up the Delaware, and called in Dr. Hutchinson to help persuade Mrs. Biddle to leave. That good lady refused to budge without her husband. Almost afraid to let the Doctor approach with his infected, vinegar-soaked clothes, Biddle nevertheless admitted him to his parlor.

Hutchinson's three days of enquiring had taught him much. He no longer scoffed at Rush's warnings, but said plainly to both his friends that there was a dangerous fever in town and they had best leave it. Then, taking Biddle aside where his wife could not hear, the large, kindly Doctor added that he had never seen anything so alarming, and urged Biddle to depart at once. "He said, that as a physician he thought it his duty to remain, and let the disorder be ever so bad, he would not leave town."

Biddle walked a little way down the street with Hutchinson, and as they separated the Doctor gravely offered his hand, saying he doubted they would ever meet again. They never did.

On Sunday afternoon, trudging through the fury of the northeast storm, Dr. Hutchinson made his way to State House Yard. He entered the little building of the American Philosophical Society and climbed up the stairs to the chamber of the College of Physicians. The Fellows were gathering. It was an extraordinary thing, this special meeting the Mayor had requested. It was the first time the city had ever asked the Fellows a sheerly medical question. Indeed, it was the first time in American history any organized medical society had been appealed to by a government, and the Fellows were sensible of their responsibilities. The city expected leadership from them, and decision, and encouragement—expected whatever help the best of medical science could give.

And it was the best of medical science the Fellows represented. They were citizen-doctors, moral, political, and social leaders, entirely competent to direct the whole community in civic action programs.

Of all the doctors in the city, the twenty-six Fellows of the College were the specialists, the teachers, the lecturers. They were vested medical authority. Not all of them turned up that Sunday afternoon. No one expected Dr. Redman, the venerable president; but Leib, Glentworth, Harris, Waters, Foulke, and others might have come. They could have told of fever cases, they might have helped Hutchinson answer the Governor's questions.

Still, the sixteen who did come were the great leaders, the scientists and practitioners who had made Philadelphia America's medical center. Shippen arrived, and as vice-president would preside, an elegant, contentious, able, devious man, brilliant professor of anatomy, midwifery, and surgery at the University, strange combination of genius and worldly vanity. And Griffitts came—Samuel Powel Griffitts, the College's secretary, gentle Quaker, dull professor, tireless in good works, a slight, gray little person, soft-spoken, hard-working, penurious, highly successful in practice, accustomed to reading the New Testament every day in Latin or Greek.

Benjamin Say, the treasurer, was no professor; indeed, he was scarcely trained in medicine at all. But he had a large practice, was wealthy and popular, a public figure, principal backer of John Fitch's steamboat enterprises, horticulturist, and abolitionist. No theorist, but an apt pupil of his learned brethren, Say could easily be impressed by their learning.

Adam Kuhn, meticulous, precise, lantern-jawed, dogmatic, protégé of Shippen, pupil of the great Linnaeus, professor of the practice of physic in the University and skillful botanist—Kuhn, respected though not loved, attended. So did Parke and Wistar, both the Duffields, Gibbons, Ross, Carson, M'Ilvaine, Dorsey, Rush, and Currie—Rush with his fixed opinions, Currie with a thoughtful dissent.

Dr. William Currie, of all those present, was the least prepared to accept Rush's pronouncements, the best prepared to refute them. Currie could cite medical authority and practice from much of the world in support of his arguments. Son of an Episcopal clergyman of Chester, learned in Latin, Greek, and Hebrew, army surgeon in the Revolution, well known for his strenuous efforts to popularize vaccination, Currie was at the height of his career. He had studied under Dr. Kearsley and practiced in Chester until 1787, when he had removed to Philadelphia and become one of the founders of the College of Physicians.

Neither teacher nor professor, Currie had about him no such

multitude of students and followers as surrounded Shippen, Griffitts, Kuhn, Hutchinson, and Rush. He also lacked their public reputation, for except for signing a temperance memorial of the College in 1787 he had stayed out of political affairs. But in the science of medicine itself he had won a distinguished place by his writing, on the very subject, actually, that the College was considering that afternoon. He had published *A Dissertation on the Autumnal Remitting Fever,* and a more substantial work, *An Historical Account of the Climates and Diseases of the United States of America.* Currie was quite prepared to admit there was fever abroad, but that it was anything more than the usual summer complaint he had serious doubts.

These sixteen physicians, collected together, as Griffitts noted in the minutes, in "Special Meeting in consequence of the prevalence of a fever of a very alarming nature in some parts of the city," began to consider "what steps should be taken by them on the occasion consistent with their duty to their fellow citizens."

Now for the study of an epidemic these sixteen gentleman-scientists of the College of Physicians were not particularly well equipped, their principal handicap being the fact that they were gentleman-scientists. Epidemics are facts, not theories. They are most appreciated by those who see them earliest, and know them best. Such people were not the Fellows; they were those other practitioners of physic of all levels who served the city.

In Philadelphia dozens of quacks and empirics plied their various trades. Midwives and nurses, barber-surgeons, dentists, aurists, cancer doctors, apothecaries, soothsayers, wandering healers salved the physical and psychic ills of the poor for a small fee. They saw epidemic disorders first. Not all their ideas were bad, as Benjamin Rush often said, and in truth not all empirics were charlatans. James Gardette, for example, surgeon-dentist, was a sensible young Frenchman who had been in this country fifteen years. He had already conceived some of his mechanical inventions in dentistry, and was skillfully constructing false teeth. And the profession of surgeon-barber had gained some respectability. The Philip Clumbergs, father and son, and Frederick and David Hailer were established bleeders to two generations. They were useful and active citizens. So were John Wharton, Godfrey Wesler, and that William Trautwine, "surgeon-barber and hair powder manufacturer" whom Rush recommended as bleeder to his patients.

An empiric, though a sterling character, was Dr. Say's father, old Thomas Say, harness maker and apothecary. He was trustee of the Negro school, manager of the Almshouse, a saintly Quaker admired about the city for his benevolent disposition and his enchanting visions. Friend Say related his visions in First Day Meeting with prodigious spiritual effect. He prescribed medicines to the poor who flocked to his chemist's shop, he performed, his son the doctor declared, "many cures, which the learned professor would not be ashamed to acknowledge." He healed by the power of sympathy—removed wens and glandular tumors simply by stroking his hands over them, and once Dr. Say saw him cure a woman of fits.

Such people were closer to the fever than the Fellows of the College. They could have supplied significant facts from their observations, had they possessed the instincts and habits of science.

Nor were the sixteen doctors assembled truly representative of Philadelphia professional opinion. The College was an exclusive organization, dedicated to the improvement of medical science. It was distinguished and famous, but it was also somewhat removed from the common run of men. There were no less than eighty physicians in the city in 1793, and many more lived and practiced in the environs. Some of those outside the College were men of importance—Dr. George Logan of Stenton, for example, Dr. Hugh Hodge, and General Washington's personal physician Dr. Samuel Bard. Dr. Frederic Phile, naval officer of the port for many years, young Thomas Hewson, who had been at Passy with Franklin, and Dr. James Graham were not Fellows, but were respectable medical men.

Some of the town's doctors were admittedly curious people. John Sparhawk was a "physician and bookseller." Mistress Hannah Toy of South Third Street described herself as "doctress." A good number were both "physician and apothecary," a combination of employments not always undignified, for such men as Amos Gregg and John Leybert were fully qualified and trained doctors, though they mixed and sold medicines. And the Frenchman David Nassy called himself "physician and druggist," but he was a member of the Philosophical Society and was amply to demonstrate his medical skill this plague year.

The doctors were scattered all through the city. Any street as far out as Sixth had its share of offices and waiting rooms. Dr. Phile and several others lived even beyond that. In Front Street half a dozen, and more than a dozen up and down Second Street, served the busiest parts of town. In Second Street old Redman lived, and Hutchinson and Nassy and Benjamin Say; so did Fiss, Goss, Harris, Janus, Perkins, Sparhawk, Weaver, and several others.

The younger men were not Fellows, though many had some contact with the College through continual conference with the professors under whom they had studied. Thus Woodhouse in Southwark, John Porter, John Penington, James Mease, William Annan, and other former students were eyes and ears for Rush as they went about the city. Some, like Woodhouse and Mease, would eventually win fame. But most of the physicians of 1793 were men who left no record but their names, who influenced little if at all the opinions of the Fellows. Dr. George F. Alberti was described by a contemporary as "gentle, soft-spoken, affectionate and profane," but of Christie, Conover, Keelmle, M'Crea, Norgrave, Pfeiffer George and Pfeiffer Joseph, Sarneighysen, Reynolds, Sloan—of men like these we know only names and addresses. Five dozen such were in the city. One Thornton called himself doctor, at Callowhill and Ridge Road, but beyond that he is gone from memory.

Even less in touch with the College were refugee physicians

from the West Indies. One of these was originally American, Dr. Edward Stevens of St. Croix, but he was better known to politicians than physicians; and as for the French and Santo Domingans, they lived isolated from all but men like Stephen Girard who could speak their tongue. Some of these French doctors had brilliant careers behind them. Some had come from the great French schools which Philadelphians (trained at Edinburgh and London, steeped in their Cullenian and Brunonian theories) knew of only vaguely. Some, like LaRoche, Devèze, and Mongés, were to move on from the fever of 1793 to great eminence, but most of the Fellows of the College of Physicians never ceased to regard them as eccentric and uninformed foreigners who practiced a barbarous technique.

The sixteen Fellows, therefore, were not really in the best position to describe the fever, nor were they the best men to do so. They were, however, an impressive company, who carried much of the load of Philadelphia's civic enterprise, and to whom the respectable and influential orders of society would listen. The College's purposes were to advance the science of medicine, to cultivate order and uniformity in the practice of physic. The Fellows were apt to these designs, busy public men who ran the medical institutions of the city.

They ran the Pennsylvania Hospital, the Philadelphia Dispensary, the medical department of the University. They sat on boards of private charitable institutions like Christ Church Hospital for aged Episcopal women and the Friends' Almshouse for Quakers who had "fallen into decay." They were managers of that unique Philadelphia organization, "The Humane Society for Recovering Persons from Suspended Animation &c." The "Suspended Animation &c." was originally drowning, but not enough persons drowned each year to use up the funds, so the Humane Society also recovered persons from heat, cold, damps, and lightning, from suffocation by charcoal, drinking cold water, and similar disasters. Grapples and apparatus had been placed at the eleven ferries on both rivers and at various shops around the city, and whenever a case of suspended animation was detected people would send at once for Rush, Wistar, Glentworth, or Say.

The Abolition Society, the Temperance Society, the various national societies, the political and social clubs, the Masonic orders, the Society of the Cincinnati, churches, and all useful or ornamental endeavors that required management found Fellows of the College in positions of leadership. For to be a Fellow was to be at the top of the medical profession. The American Philosophical Society was twenty-five years old, and for twenty-five years Dr. Adam Kuhn had been an officer. Barton and Wistar were curators, Griffitts, Rush, and Hutchinson were councilors, doctors were frequent participants in its sessions.

Rush was in everything. Griffitts was in everything Quaker. Hutchinson was in everything Republican, Shippen in everything fashionable.

II

It was more than natural, it was inevitable, that such men should disagree. Not on the facts, to be sure, but on the theory. All were ready to answer *yes* to the first question, was there a malignant fever abroad in the city? But on the other questions— where did it come from? how was it spread?—the Fellows discovered profound differences. They spent the afternoon, Griffitts wrote, in "a free communication of sentiment," exploring the old argument, was fever imported and contagious, or domestic and carried in the fouled solids of the air?

It was the theory of the thing the Fellows worried about. No one described cases, for a case was interesting only if it proved a theory. The essence of medicine was theory, principle, rational understanding. The healing art had to be studied systematically. Obviously there were only so many diseases in the world, and obviously they all had to be catalogued and classified. Illustrious Dr. Cullen of Edinburgh had given every disease its place in a great taxonomy of ills, just as Linnaeus had arranged all plants in phylums. First, there were the big Classes of diseases; then each Class had its various Orders, each Order several Genera, each Genus many Species. Nosology, the doctors called this classification of diseases. It was nosology that made the difference between empirics and true physicians. Empirics, ignorant of the class and order and species of a disease, of its remote and proximate causes, ignorant of all nosology, treated only the grossest symptoms, not the real root of illness. Their practice was habit, founded in caprice and continued in ignorance, however they might dignify it with the name of experience. But the true physician reflected on the nature and causes of disease. He exercised his understanding.

It was just like thunder and lightning, Currie said. The effects of thunder and lightning had been known long before Dr. Franklin's time, but until Franklin discovered their nature and causes, no one ever thought "of the means by which they might be disarmed of their destructive power."

The only trouble was, theory left such immense room for disagreement. On the nosology of fever there were two completely different theories. Currie followed Dr. Cullen's nosology: all fevers belonged to Class I of disease; Class I had five different Orders in it, each Order numerous Genera, each Genus several Species of fever, each Species its own special causes and symptoms. Autumnal remittent was a Species belonging to one Genus in one Order, typhus gravior to another, bilious camp fever to a third, scarlet fever to a fourth. The malignant yellow fever—Currie called it *synochus icteroides*—belonged still elsewhere. The yellow fever had its special and particular causes. By Currie's nosology it was of foreign origin, and propagated only by contagion. One sick person gave it to others. It was just the disease one would expect from the influx of the Santo Domingans.

Rush, on the other hand, had abandoned his teacher Cullen, and developed a nosology all his own. Rush believed that all fevers were one and the same fever, that all had one cause. Since the only thing everybody shared in common was the air they breathed, the causative factor of fever had to exist in the air.

Anyone, Santo Domingans and Philadelphians alike, could receive contagion from putrified air.

To every doctor, whatever his nosology, the great mystery of the air around him made a strong appeal. Imagination filled the aether with all kinds of fluids and solids, gave it all sorts of qualities, feared all manner of dangers lurking in it. Air contained the vital principle of life itself. What disease was not affected by the unknown, unknowable chemistry of the air?

Even contagionists like Currie admitted that infections were "strengthened by a particular construction of the atmosphere." Dry weather and putrefaction destroyed "oxygen gas or pure air," Currie wrote, and thereby nurtured diseases. But this was only an influence—the air could not actually start infection. All that talk about rotting coffee and decaying animal matter was nonsense, he felt, for though such stuff smelled bad, it only gave off a little "hydrogen gas or inflammable air" slightly different from growing grass or live vegetables.

Other theorists went farther than this. They pointed to the many cemeteries in Philadelphia, from which the rays of the sun drew up continual fetid exhalations, imperceptible perhaps, but most certainly there. And they saw air passing over putrid coffee, stinking wharves, dirty markets. These foul influences, Dr. David Nassy believed, "added to the quantity of vapours, and of corpuscles of all kinds with which the atmosphere is always loaded, cannot but rarify or thicken the liquids, affect the solids, and derange the animal economy in the most sensible manner."

Only three things could clear the air, Nassy declared—the three purifying agents, wind and rain and thunder. Yet in the long drought Philadelphia had seen none of these for many weeks. The city was still breathing last June's air. No wonder infections flourished.

But Dr. Rush's view was otherwise. He believed "the sensible and insensible qualities of the air" actually caused fevers, and he accounted for the thirty years' absence of yellow fever by saying that Philadelphia's air was changing lately. He had written a little book about it: *An Account of the Climate of Pennsylvania, and Its Influence on the Human Body.* He showed how social progress changed the atmosphere: how when the British army had cut the trees between the city and the Schuylkill, for example, fevers had come immediately in that region, how they had ceased (oddly enough) as soon as the cleared land was turned under the plow. Every time a gristmill was built, fevers resulted. They appeared only on the west side of the milldam—because, Rush guessed, the prevailing winds which carried the exhalations were easterly. Years before, fevers had been confined to the shores of rivers in Pennsylvania, "but since the country has been so much cleared of woods, we often meet with them eight or ten miles from the rivers."

The climatic changes, he decided, were not easy to describe, because of the variability of Pennsylvania's weather from year to year. "There are no two successive years alike. . . . Perhaps there is but one steady trait in the character of our climate, and that is, it is uniformly variable." It was, he decided, "a compound of most of the climates of the world."

This variability of the climate did not, he thought, make Pennsylvania *"necessarily* unhealthy"—indeed, the air of the Commonwealth had a "peculiar elasticity, which renders the heat and cold less insupportable than the same degree of both are in moister countries." And dikes, drainage ditches, the paving of Dock Creek, and such things had converted Philadelphia from "the most sickly, to one of the healthiest cities in the United States."

Thus, Rush considered, it had been proved, that cleaning up filth could remove pollution of the air which caused fevers. But about those great mysterious forces at work in the climate, those dimly perceived alterations in the whole atmosphere, mere men could do nothing at all.

Traditions as old as medicine itself lay behind the opinions Rush, Currie, and the other Fellows had formed. Thucydides and Herodotus, Hippocrates and Galen were part of their thinking. So were the "greats" of modern medicine—Sydenham,

Boerhaave, Cullen, Monro, Lettsom, Brown. Sydenham had argued a century ago that fever was not itself a disease, but only a manifestation of disease. And nearly everyone conceded by now that the heat of the body in fevers was a material substance separate from the body—perhaps the same substance that was carried by the infected air. Some authorities were even saying that fever was not an affection "of this or that humour alone" but of the whole body, and therefore a disease apart.

But from the lecture halls of Edinburgh young graduates in medicine had gone out to all corners of the world taking with them the doctrines of Cullen and Monro. Fevers, Cullen had said, were contagious. He had not talked about fetid miasmas or putrified solids of the air. He had talked about the dangers of sick people. Contagion he defined as "effluvia arising directly or originally from the body of a man under a particular disease, and exciting the same kind of disease in the body of the person to whom they are applied." For most doctors, this was the leading thought on contagion; it was the rule of natural law which young Britishers took with them to distant places where they saw fevers in action.

They observed fevers everywhere through Cullen's eyes, wrote books about them in their teacher's words. Whole shelves of these books were available to Philadelphia doctors, and exciting reading they made. There was Chisholm on West India fevers, Cleghorn on *Diseases of Minorca,* Russell on a plague at Aleppo, Jackson, Hunter, and others on fevers in Jamaica, Sir John Pringle's *Diseases of the Army* (which covered every climate in the Empire), and several works by the lively Dr. James Lind—one on fevers in Bengal, another *On the Diseases Incidental to Europeans in Hot Climates.* There were many more. The eighteenth-century world seemed literally ridden with fevers, and everyone had its Cullenian chronicler. For Philadelphians who hoped that fevers came from tropical climates, these books furnished ample proof.

And a good many Americans had described fevers too, even before Currie's recent publications. The first clinical lecture ever given in America had been Dr. Thomas Bond's in Philadelphia in 1766—he had devoted it to the yellow fever. The great Cadwallader Colden of New York had written on the subject, Dr. John Kearsley of Philadelphia produced an essay, Dr. Walton of Boston published a work on *Fever, the Rattles, and Canker;* in Virginia Dr. John Mitchell kept careful notes on the plagues of 1737 and 1742 and eventually sent them to Benjamin Franklin.

If the Fellows had only known it, one American book argued against Cullen in favor of Rush. It was by John Moultrie, Jr., of South Carolina, called *De Febre Maligna Biliosa Americæ.* Moultrie had written and published it as a dissertation at Edinburgh in the 1740's, and later it was edited and republished in Europe by Professor Boldenger of Jena, who pronounced it the best existing account of yellow fever. It was well known in Europe, but strangely never published in America. Probably no Philadelphia doctor knew it. Had they, Rush might have won his point, for Moultrie contended that fever was caused locally by marsh effluvia, violent exercise, excessive drinking, and the heat of the air.

All the Fellows knew another American book, however: the *History of the Yellow Fever* by John Lining of Charleston, which the College of Physicians declared was the best description of the disease. Lining was a Cullenian contagionist. He believed in West India origin, had fixed the conviction firmly in American thinking. And in Charleston another doctor, Lionel Chalmers, had also written on fevers—written several books, all to the same effect as Lining's.

Most of the weight of authority seemed against Rush's ideas about the coffee, the markets, the foul smells, and the filth of the city. Most medical opinion favored importation, contagion, and quarantine. And the Santo Domingans seemed to clinch it. Certainly one could not dismiss them; certainly everyone heard they had brought sickness with them.

Yet there were conflicting reports, even about that. Dr. Jean Devèze, for example, had been a passenger on that twice-captured brig *Mary* from Cap François to Philadelphia, and Dr. Devèze insisted that far from being feverish, the crowded vessel had carried only three persons ill of any disease—two ladies who showed no yellow fever symptoms, and another who had a miscarriage. As for the *Sans Culottes*, Devèze contended the captain and surgeon reported no sick on board, though it had been said around the city that the captain himself and some of his crew had died.

Fortunately, perhaps, Devèze's firsthand information regarding the *Mary* and his strange confidence concerning the *Sans Culottes* did not reach the College—fortunately, because the Fellows already had enough confusing evidence and contradictory theory to deal with in their "free communication of sentiment." They must perforce reach a conclusion.

Everyone spoke his mind; then a committee was appointed "to consider and report on the means best adapted to prevent the spreading of this disease and to guard against the contagion of it." Rush, Hutchinson, Say, and Wistar were named, and directed to have their report ready next day. These four consulted together, and asked Dr. Rush to prepare their report. At once Rush walked home through the rain and sat down to write it. He labored far into the night.

Next day—Monday, August 26—the College met again to hear Rush's report. Only eleven Fellows came this time. They adopted the report unanimously, and sent it to the Mayor. Clarkson in turn relayed it to the Governor, to congressmen and legislators, and then had it published in the papers. Their principal task accomplished, the less-than-a-dozen Fellows resolved that the College should continue to meet, "every Monday at 4 P.M. to confer upon the treatment of the existing malignant fever during its prevalence in this city."

To the people the Fellows offered little comfort. They had found no sure preventive, no certain cure; nor did they minimize the danger. The report spoke brutally of "the malignant and contagious fever, which now prevails." The words "yellow fever" were not mentioned, nor was the filth and pollution about the city given as the cause. Anyone looking for hope might have found it in these omissions. But no sensible person, reading the report, could miss the fearful apprehensions of the doctors.

Yet at least the Fellows offered a program. The report suggested things to do, and things not to do. It treated the disorder as a problem to be met. This was leadership of a sort. Eleven measures the College proposed to the citizens, and to the whole city—eleven measures of prevention and protection:

Avoid every infected person, as much as possible.

Avoid fatigue of body and mind. Don't stand or sit in a draft, or in the sun, or in the evening air.

Dress according to the weather. Avoid intemperance. Drink sparingly of wine, beer, or cider.

When visiting the sick, use vinegar or camphor on your handkerchief, carry it in smelling bottles, use it frequently.

Somehow mark every house with sickness in it, on the door or window.

Place your patients in the center of your biggest, airiest room, in beds without curtains. Change their clothes and bed linen often. Remove all offensive matter as quickly as possible.

Stop the tolling of the bells at once.

Bury the dead in closed carriages, as privately as possible.

Clean the streets, and keep them clean.

Stop building fires in your houses, or on the streets. They have no useful effect. But burn gunpowder. It clears the air. And use vinegar and camphor generally.

Most important of all, let a large and airy hospital be provided near the city, to receive poor people stricken with the disease who cannot otherwise be cared for.

Now this seemed to cover most of the points people had been debating all week, but the report, significantly, said nothing about Santo Domingans. Neither did Dr. Hutchinson, in the letter he composed answering the Governor. The popular Hutchinson was obviously confused. First he had denied there was a fever, then changed his mind. Next he had said around the city that the French ships had brought it, now he refrained from mentioning them. Clearly Hutchinson had been influenced by the College's free communication of sentiment. His answer to Governor Mifflin revealed how much.

Hutchinson stated bluntly that a malignant fever had certainly appeared, and was spreading. He noted that Dr. Say had seen cases in Kensington before the outbreak in Water Street, which if correct would contradict the theory of the putrid coffee. He estimated that forty deaths had occurred—Rush said the number was really above a hundred and fifty—but he added that he had heard of no foreigners or sailors infected.

He concluded boldly, "It does not appear to be an imported disease."

Foulke, had he bothered to attend the meeting, could have told the Fellows of stricken foreigners and sailors. So could young Cathrall or Physick or the French physicians. But the College, isolated in its professional dignities, had discovered no reason to quarantine the West India refugees.

Hutchinson was Port Physician. He should have walked down to the docks. But the huge and amiable Dr. Hutchinson was not feeling very well.

Prevention, Personal and Civic

AUGUST 27–31

. . . humanly speaking, had decisive measures been
adopted any time before the first of September,
while the disorder existed only in one street, and
in a few houses in that street, there can be little
doubt, that it might have been very soon extin-
guished.—MATHEW CAREY

ON the dockside, in Front Street, along Second and Third, in
Kensington, Southwark, in the city's little alleys—in Appletree
and Black Horse, Blackberry, Brooke's Court, Elbow Lane and
Elfreth's Alley—in Letitia Court, Laurel and Mulberry, in
Pewter-platter Alley, Sassafras and Scheibell's, Strawberry,
Sugar and Whalebone—in all crowded districts, people were
sickening now. Tragedies of the first week were forgotten in
the far greater disasters of the second.

On Monday, August 26, the rain stopped. The northeast
wind continued, the clouds hovered, but the barometer gradually
rose. It was damp and sultry. Through the muddy streets that
day seventeen bodies were carried to the graveyards—three to
the Catholic, four to the Lutheran, two to Christ Church, people
counted the frightening train and slammed down their windows
as the coffins passed. Before their hearths, they sat listening to
the mournful tolling of the bells.

On Tuesday, citizens lit fires again at street corners, to
purify the rain-soaked air. That day the College's report was
published, and at once the church bells were stilled, as the report
recommended. The great silence began. Continual ringing hour

after hour had terrorized the sick and depressed the well, yet
the great silence was even worse. It was a confession of defeat.

The weather cleared that week as August drew to a close. The
heats came back, funerals mounted. On Wednesday there were
twenty-two, on Thursday twenty-four, Friday twenty, on Saturday, August 31, seventeen. John Dunkin, aged twenty-five, one
of the city's bright and eligible young men, was buried on
Wednesday, not privately as the College had urged but with a
large train of mourners. The deaths of John Morgan, merchant,
and "Mrs. Ann Comegys consort of Mr. Comegys merchant"
were noted in the papers. By Saturday, thirty-eight people in
eleven families in Water Street had died—all in the space of nine
days. Rush lost five patients on the twenty-sixth, and expected
five more to die that night. He noted the departure of the Chews,
the Lewises, Dr. White's family: "Our neighbourhood will be
desolate in a day or two," he told his wife.

The College's report had immediate effect. While a visitor in
the city on Sunday had heard nothing of a plague, after Tuesday
the twenty-seventh no one doubted that a general pestilence was
abroad. At once the very appearance of the street changed.
People stayed indoors scouring, whitewashing, "purifying"
their houses, burning gunpowder, tobacco, and nitre, sprinkling
vinegar. Those who had to walk abroad carried their tarred
ropes or camphor bags and chewed garlic constantly, doused
themselves with vinegar, carried smelling bottles or smoked
tobacco. They emitted a curious odor for several yards. Even
women and small boys, Mathew Carey observed, had segars
almost constantly in their mouths, and remedies by the dozen
were concocted. It was said that Dr. Hutchinson was weak from
inhaling camphor and debilitating scents.

People quickly acquired the habits of living with fear. Hand-
shaking was abandoned, acquaintances snubbed, everyone
walked in the middle of the streets to avoid contaminated houses.
Those wearing mourning bands were obviously dangerous, as
were doctors and ministers. People maneuvered in passing to
get to windward of anyone they met. Watches and clocks in the

city went madly off, but there were no clockmakers to fix them. One night the watch called all the hours wrong.

Vain attempts were made to quiet public fears. Andrew Brown, editor of the *Federal Gazette,* published all the Mayor's impressive orders, the Governor's letters, and heartening notices. One day he even announced in a conspicuous place, "from the assurances of several respectable Physicians" that the fever was considerably abated. But it was a foolish thing to say, and he did not again try to disguise the truth. People were all too well apprised of the disease, by its own appearance and action. It was, Friend Susan Dillwyn wrote tremulously, a time of such anxiety and distress as was never before known in America.

Business processes collapsed unexpectedly. So many seamen were sick that ships lay tied up at the docks, and incoming vessels could find no wharfage.

All the schools in town suddenly closed, some because teachers ordered it, others because scholars deserted. Servants feared to go outside the house, even to draw water from the pump. "Dejection sits on every countenance," Rush wrote. He hoped his report for the College would do some good, but he knew nothing would really subdue the fever before the heavy rains or frosts of October.

The northeast storm, for some reason, had not cleared the air. Perhaps it was because the source of infection was still about. Dr. John Foulke, who had not bothered to attend the College's meeting, had occupied himself instead on Sunday writing a letter to Mayor Clarkson. Foulke was worried about that coffee. He observed that a whole week had gone by since the "discovery," yet there on Joseph Ball's Wharf the coffee still sat, foul and putrid in a stinking heap. Since he lived within sight and smell of the offensive stuff, Foulke regarded it with special distaste.

Whether because of the coffee or not, air which the great force of a northeaster could not purge must be fouled indeed. Dr. Rush asked his wife to stay in Princeton with the youngest children, but he had the three older sons (as well as his mother and sister) at home with him. The boys feared to touch him or get near his clothes when he came in from visiting patients. By and by they complained of headaches, so he packed them off to Trenton. He advised everyone who could to leave the city. There was only one certain preventive of the disease—"Fly from it!"

Rush waxed more fearful every day, for the fever grew stranger with every case. It defied all medicine, it even defied the understanding. Everyone, sick or well, seemed apathetic and lazy. One of Rush's patients, Mr. Stiles the stonecutter, exhibited symptoms of the true plague before he died—those buboes or large carbuncles, hard, balled swellings with black apexes which discharged a thin, dark-colored bloody matter. All the doctors feared these signs. They had seen them during the Revolutionary War in army camp fevers; now they watched apprehensively as the buboes appeared again. Such symptoms did not, Rush thought, mean the disease was really the true plague; but what they did mean was beyond him.

Some cases began with violent chills and temperatures, others with languor and nausea. Stupor, delirium, vomit, slow pulse, bloodshot eyes, yellowness regularly succeeded. Sometimes patients remained sensible and conscious to the last. One man shaved himself just before he died. "Livid spots on the body"— those inexplicable eruptions which "resembled moscheto bites" —"a bleeding at the nose, from the gums and from the bowels, and a vomiting of black matter in some instances close the scenes of life," Rush recorded.

All known remedies failed. The only things Rush found helpful were wrapping the patients in hot vinegar-soaked blankets and dousing them with cold water. He consulted constantly with Dr. Wistar and derived, he declared, "great support and assistance from him in all my attempts to stop the progress of this terrible malady." Wistar he thought "an excellent man," who rose "in his humanity and activity with the danger and distress of his fellow citizens."

By the middle of this second week Dr. Rush was frantic with worry and exhausted by calls upon him. His mother, sister, and assistants were devoted to his comfort; they stretched a mattress across some chairs on which he could lie and rest for a few minutes every time he came into the house, without having to go near the other rooms. Late Tuesday night he wrote, "In mercy to my fellow citizens and family, my life so long and so often forfeited to divine justice, is *still* preserved." Thursday night he told his wife, "Be assured that I will send for you, if I should be seized with the disorder, for I conceive that it would be as much your duty not to desert me in that situation, as it is now mine not to desert my patients." And early Friday he added a postscript: "Aug: 30th. Another night and morning have been added to my life. I am preparing to sett off for my daily round of duty, and feel heartily disposed to say with Jabez, 'O that the hand of the Lord may be with me' not only to preserve my life, but to heal my poor patients."

II

Ebenezer Hazard was no doctor. He was, as a matter of fact, secretary of the Insurance Company of North America. It was a good job, and he was proud of it; but he had many other interests as well. He had promoted canals and bridges, had been Postmaster-General, lately he had blossomed into literary scholarship. He was hard at work on the second volume of his *Historical Collections*. From his "snug, retired room" he observed the strange disorder and followed all the steps Mayor Clarkson was taking with special interest, for the Mayor was his mother's brother. Some thought the fever imported, he wrote, or caused by the crowding of the vessels from Cap François. Others thought it arose from the dry, sultry season and absence of thunder. Hazard leaned to the latter solution, and he had a speculation of his own to contribute: perhaps the large number of lightning rods fixed to houses in the city (one of Dr. Franklin's lesser legacies), "by imperceptibly drawing off the electric fluid from the clouds, and thereby preventing thunder," contributed to the increase of disease.

It was conceivable. Anything was conceivable, for nothing was sure or certain about this fantastic sickness. Basic medical questions confronted the doctors, unsolved. For example, what exactly was that black vomit? No one knew. One doctor said it was putrid bile, another putrid blood. A third pronounced it the villous coating of the stomach thrown up as the innards disintegrated. A fourth thought it simple bile turned black because it encountered nitric acid in the stomach and intestines. Or it may have originated in the kidneys, or liver, or spleen. Dr. Stevens and Dr. Physick said it was the result of disease in the stomach. Since it came in the last stages of the fever, everyone regarded it as terribly infectious and dangerous. Even young Dr. Cathrall, who had seen it analyzed, was unwilling to touch the stuff. At Edinburgh in 1792 he had sat under Dr. Monro, who showed his class a vial of black vomit sent him from the West Indies. Monro had not let the vial out of his hands, however, so Cathrall acquired only a respectful theoretical acquaintance with the substance. For him and all the other physicians the loathsome, putrid vomit remained a frightening aspect of the disease.

Nor did the great variety of symptoms help the doctors understand their problem. Some were not yet ready to accept Rush's diagnosis. Though the College said publicly that its report had been unanimously adopted and published it as an official collective recommendation, many in the city knew that Rush had written it, and that very few doctors had attended the meetings. Some viewed the report with suspicion as the production of a highly contentious individual and his partisans.

A physician writing as "Quaestor Veritatis" challenged it. Taking Currie's line, he stated that the malady was not the yellow fever, but only a modified form of the influenza or epidemic catarrh, which everyone knew had been increasing. Debilitated by the unusual summer heat and drought, the inhabitants were more susceptible to fever than ever before. That Water Street appeared the center of infection was not the result of some local source of contagion. Rather, it resulted from the fact that the air was less pure there. Water Street houses were half buried under the ground, and "the quantity of filth and stagnant water, excrementous substances in a state of putrefaction" in the little street not only confined the air, but robbed it of "its vivifying principle, for want of which, fire cannot be kindled, nor animals breathe."

"Quaestor" also said the College's proposal to mark infected houses was cruel and unnecessary, giving sanction "to an opinion of the plague being among us." No one would visit houses so marked; wretched sufferers would perish for want of help; marketing and commercial intercourse along the wharves would cease.

"Quaestor Veritatis" was not the only objector. Every Philadelphian by now was talking of the fever. Chemists were advertising Peruvian bark, salt of vinegar, refined camphor, and other "elegant compositions" for preventing infection. Daffey's Elixir, a preparation so highly alcoholic that it intoxicated when it did not purge, was a favorite tonic. A new physician, Dr. William Barnwell, who averred he had had much experience with the disorders of warm climates, offered his services at 87 South Third Street (just around the corner from Rush's) "at this alarming and critical period." The many citizens who had been kindling fires in front of their houses and on street corners, filling the city with smoke and ashes, were not deterred by the College's report that fires would do no good. So dangerous were the flames, however, and such a nuisance, that Mayor Clarkson ordered the practice stopped, citing Rush's report to convince the frightened people.

Just then a remedy promising even more danger was suggested—the discharging of cannon, which would clear the air. It was a device "the late Dr. Chevot, who for a great number of years lived in the West Indies" was said to have advocated, and a helpful citizen indicated that the artillery company would probably be glad of the exercise.

In the midst of tension the Pennsylvania legislature met, assembling in the State House at three in the afternoon of Tuesday, August 27. If all else failed, the plague could be legislated out of existence. In their noble chamber in Independence

Hall, ten of the eighteen senators were called to order by Speaker Samuel Powel, thirty-eight (about half) of the representatives arrived. It was a routine session, but even on the second day, before the Governor's formal speech, a bill was introduced calling for an amendment of the health laws. The third day, Thursday, August 29, found the representatives distinctly uneasy. A young man named Joseph Fry, their doorkeeper, occupied an apartment in the west wing of the State House, and Joseph Fry, they learned that day, lay dead in his rooms of the fever. Acutely conscious of his nearness to their hall, the representatives passed a resolution, that *whereas* a malignant and contagious fever was abroad in the city, and *whereas* it existed near the State House, and *whereas* to assemble large numbers of people in one room might spread the infection, *now therefore* let the Governor be requested to send his message in writing. This resolution the smaller Senate in its larger room disdainfully voted down, and the gentlemen of the House were forced to troop in, reeking of vinegar and camphor. Governor Mifflin was introduced, seated in the speaker's chair, and proceeded to read his address.

His Excellency had a good many things to say on the state of the Union and of Pennsylvania. He talked of the war in Europe, and of American neutrality with all its problems; of prize ships and privateers, of the fortifications around Philadelphia and in the Delaware River, of the Pennsylvania militia, the national Indian War in Ohio and negotiations for a treaty, of the finances of the state; he referred to the Santo Domingans and their relief. Then he added a final paragraph urging the improvement of the health office. This office, he observed, "becomes daily more important to the well being of our metropolis." Too astute to assign a local origin to the disease, which might harm Philadelphia's commerce, too wily to repeat Dr. Hutchinson's categorical statement that the fever did not appear to be an imported one, the Governor spoke obliquely of the pestilence as "an infectious disorder; which, together with recent occurrences, that have increased our intercourse with the

West Indies, and the influx of foreigners, must point out the necessity of more strongly guarding the public health, by legislative precautions."

Mifflin was going to lay the plague at the Frenchmen's door if he could, regardless of what the College said. He had, he assured the legislature, instituted proper enquiries, and was confident that "the Health Officer, and the Physician of the Port, aided by the Officers of the Police, and the Gentlemen of the Faculty," would pursue "every rational measure to allay the public inquietude, and effectually remove its cause.

Whether the Governor really felt such confidence on Thursday the twenty-ninth was of no account; what he obviously did feel was the immediate need for a public display of spirit. Returning from the legislative halls to his office, he wrote out a sharp, gratuitously critical letter to Mayor Clarkson, preparing a copy for the newspapers. Professing he was sorry to interfere with the Mayor's work, he enjoined vigorous measures; and he assured Clarkson the legislature would bear the expense of any necessary action the aldermen and council refused to pay for. "I do not hesitate, therefore, to desire," said Mifflin (giving the color of a fanciful official sanction to his peremptory letter), "that gunpowder, and other salutory preparations, may be flashed through the streets; and that, generally the other precautions, recommended by the College of Physicians, may be strictly observed."

With a blandness surprising in Mifflin, the Governor added that he was sure Mayor Clarkson would "readily excuse the trouble and comply with the contents" of his letter.

To Mayor Clarkson, already working with utmost energy and devotion, the Governor's assurance of money was heartily welcome, but the rest of his letter must have seemed silly and political. True enough, the Mayor had not flashed "gunpowder and other salutory preparations" through the streets, for he had been entirely too busy with more serious problems. But if the Governor wished, it could be done. Clarkson ordered it, and for one whole day, August 30, the militia company from Fort

Mifflin actually hauled a small cannon through the streets, stopping every few yards to fire. Sensible people realized this was foolish, ineffectual, and ludicrous. The noise was exceedingly trying. After one day's experiment with the method of "the late Dr. Chevot," the cannon was given up.

Important steps had been taken, however, and favorable results achieved. Clarkson determined to make them public. Late Thursday night he found time to write a reply to the Governor with a full and patient account of just what had been done. It was really quite a lot.

First, there were the clean-up orders. Mayor Clarkson knew that his publications had produced few results in six days. Consequently, he had issued three new orders on Tuesday the twenty-seventh, when he received the report of the College. One went to High Constable Alexander Carlyle, directing him to visit all wharves and report any offensive, noxious substance he found on them. A second went to Joseph Ogden and Peter Smyth ordering them to clean up the market houses, flush them with the fire engines, and see to it that the butchers scrubbed their stalls and blocks. A third ordered the commissioners to keep the streets constantly clean, not confining the scavengers to the weekly collection prescribed in the ordinance, but operating continuously, for which he assured them money would be forthcoming.

These orders Clarkson described to the Governor, and he reported progress. In two days the markets had been washed by the fire engines and otherwise cleaned. The aldermen and council had appointed a committee to confer with the Guardians of the Poor. Nitre was being burned in Water Street right then as he wrote preparatory to another cleaning in the morning, and, the Mayor added, "An Hospital in an airy and healthy place is to be provided with all expedition."

Those words "with all expedition" were sadly hopeful words, for Mayor Clarkson better than any other knew the legion of difficulties that impeded every attempt to get things done. There was no reason to recite these trials in public, particularly if doing so would give the Governor a partisan advantage. Clarkson ignored the various affronts in Mifflin's letter, achieving a good effect instead by a closing reference to the charity and sympathy of Philadelphia folk.

His answer, when published along with Mifflin's, would at least sound friendly. This was no time for factional bitterness; and anyway, the Governor had promised money.

III

What the Mayor might have said, had he cared to, was that civil government in Philadelphia was breaking down. Ten days after Rush had proclaimed the pestilence, only two days after the College's report and Dr. Hutchinson's letter had been published, the ordinary processes of administration began to fall apart. Officials were frequently ill or more frequently had fled the city; no scavengers could be hired, or anyone to do the dirty jobs at hand. The Governor might speak confidently of the officers of the police, but there were mighty few to be found, and the "Gentlemen of the Faculty" were unhappily not all as devoted as Rush, Hutchinson, and Griffitts. The energetic Mayor could not stay the disease singlehanded. Yet time and again there was no one to carry his messages, to execute his orders, even to consult and advise with him.

Councilmen left, and aldermen, judges and magistrates, clerks, brokers, chimney-sweeps and carters. Constables fled, and nurses, drivers and notaries, printers, scribes and bankers. The twenty-three night watchmen supposed to be on duty every night dwindled to a handful. Even some of the Guardians were leaving, and this was the worst of all.

The "Overseers and Guardians of the Poor" occupied a curious position in the city government. They had originated as managers of the Almshouse (or House of Employment or Betterment House or Poorhouse), a great sprawling building on Spruce Street between Tenth and Eleventh, where the paupers of the city, the Northern Liberties, and Southwark were set to work in crude manufacturing. The Overseers and Guardians had been incorporated in colonial days, and given power to lay special taxes for the care of the indigent. By 1793 they were the only official agency dealing with the poor. Six of them were Overseers, managing the Almshouse, responsible for what went on inside the institution; fourteen others were Guardians, presumably overseeing and guarding the poor outside the Almshouse in the city, the Liberties, and Southwark.

Now this was a thankless sort of job, the sort young men took at the beginning of their political, professional, or commercial careers. This August all eight Philadelphia city Guardians were youthful and relatively obscure. Their business was to locate the sick poor, see that they received attention, and keep them from becoming a public nuisance.

As the disease spread in the first and second week after Rush's announcement, the Guardians found the greatest burdens of the city falling on them, for they were the liaison between the authorities and the needy. They had to hire carters for the transport of the sick, arrange for the burial of bodies, find medical and nursing assistance. And they had to do it all with no money. Their own funds were committed to the Almshouse; Mayor Clarkson could give them little.

Actually, the city's revenues were not great. Philadelphians paid about £8,600 in taxes every year; rent charged the public markets produced about £1,200, public wharves £500, the High Street ferry over the Schuylkill around £840. With these and all other sources of revenue (including sale of manure from the streets), the total income of the city government was about £15,000. Of this, £4,000 was spent "watching and lighting the city," another £4,000 paving and cleaning the streets; the street commissioners received salaries, pumps had to be sunk and repaired, wharves and docks kept clean and in good order, clerks of the markets paid, the ferry maintained, all sorts of other things done, so that out of the whole budget there was nothing left to devote to the Guardians in sudden emergencies.

Some of the Guardians simply left the city. Others, meeting every danger, stayed at their posts day and night, like the

Mayor himself, but the work soon got beyond them. Clarkson had no one to assign to help them. The risks were awful. Scavengers, carters, and watchmen would flee rather than assist the Guardians, and drivers were impossible to find.

As people in comfortable circumstances left the city, as the fortunate ones who had farms or relatives to visit streamed out, the elements of commerce began to atrophy. Work ceased in countless shops, stores, and homes. Servants, clerks, and laborers were idle. Overnight, it seemed, the city thronged with jobless. In a day, the jobless were hungry. They added to the Guardians' problems, for they swelled the great class of the less fortunate, the poor who had neither horse nor cart nor place to go nor money to live when they got there, who had to stay penniless in the city, unable to buy medicines when they fell sick, or to fee a doctor.

The Guardians had more poor to care for than the city had ever seen, and among their poor sickness struck abundantly. Yet the Guardians had nowhere to take the indigent fever victims. Managers of institutions both public and private refused to admit them. The Guardians themselves closed the great Almshouse to the sick, under an old rule prohibiting admission of anyone with an infectious disease. More than three hundred paupers were living at the Almshouse that summer. If the fever once started there, it would be impossible to check. When two paupers, admitted with certificates of good health from doctors, died in the Almshouse of the fever, it was ordered that no more paupers at all, sick or well, should be admitted until the plague was over, though the managers offered to supply beds and bedding and all the money in their treasury for relief outside their walls.

The Pennsylvania Hospital, too, had to think of its present inmates, for it had no pesthouse. Dr. Foulke, one of the board of physicians, had actually sent two fever victims in as patients. One, a Negro, died the morning after admission; the other was in the last stages of the disease. On Wednesday, August 28, the managers met at Samuel Coates's house "for the purpose of

looking into a violation of the rules of the Hospital on account
of the patients having been admitted, said to be suffering from
'yellow fever.'" Dr. Foulke, the one who had broken the rule,
was requested to investigate the whole subject, and physicians
were asked to examine patients carefully before admitting them.

With both hospital and Almshouse barred to them, there was
no place left where the indigent, homeless ill could be cared for
—or the solitary custodians of abandoned homes, or lonely
people who lived in rented rooms, or those turned out by their
families as soon as they fell sick. In doorways and alleys, in
yards and courts, in open streets people lay dying. The Guardians of the Poor were confronted with an impossible situation.
And they were impelled by urgent necessity. Diseased paupers
were a menace to the diseased rich, and to the whole city, sick
or well. On Monday, August 26 (while the College was adopt-
ing its report), the Guardians took possession of Mr. Ricketts'
circus at Twelfth and the High.

John Bill Ricketts, the celebrated equestrian, was an enterprising Scotchman who had recently become the city's favorite
entertainer. A few months earlier he had erected an enclosed
amphitheatre out in the residential district, and there presented
his edifying spectacles before large crowds, sometimes including
President Washington himself. His fellow Scot James Hardie
described him in his *Directory* as "perhaps the most graceful,
neat, and expert public performer on horseback, that ever appeared in any part of the world. . . ." Among his many feats
were "leaping over ten horses—riding with a boy on his shoul-
der in the attitude of Mercury—going through the manuel
exercise with a firelock—dancing a hornpipe in the saddle, the
horse being in full speed, &c. &c." In short, Hardie added, the
circus was "esteemed amongst the first amusements met with
in this truly astonishing Metropolis; as a place to dispel the
gloom of the thoughtful, exercise the lively activity of the young
and gay, or to relax the minds of the sedentary or industrious
trader."

Late in July, staying his departure only long enough to play a benefit for the Santo Domingans, Ricketts had moved on to do a season in New York, obliging Philadelphia's sedentary or industrious traders to seek their relaxation elsewhere. He had left his circus at Twelfth and the High empty, and no agent remained in the city to confront the Guardians with law. They moved in.

To the circus seven stricken paupers were carried and laid in the enclosure. Through all the comfortable homes in the neighborhood their sinister presence was felt. Two of them died; the rest lay retching and vomiting day and night, cared for by no one. Somebody came and removed one of the corpses, but the other lay there among the sick more than forty-eight hours because no one would touch it. Finally the Guardians hired a carter who agreed to haul the body away, but he found he could not, singlehanded, get it into a coffin. A servant girl, "understanding the difficulties he labored under, offered her services, provided he would not inform the family with whom she lived (else she would be at once dismissed)." She helped him lift the body and force it into the box, though it was "crawling with maggots, and in the most loathsome state of putrefaction."

Now the circus was no solution at all, as everyone knew. Householders near-by were seized with terror, and threatened to burn or destroy the amphitheatre unless the repulsive sick were removed. Yet the Guardians, helpless as the problems of the week multiplied, had no other place to take them. Nor had they attendants, or nurses, or anyone willing to bury the dead.

Afterwards, Mathew Carey wrote that the want of a lazaretto where victims could be sent on first recognition of a contagious disorder had been the cause of much suffering. Decisive measures, including that hospital everyone hoped for, would have saved many lives. Decisive measures, however, required more understanding than anyone as yet possessed, required more people to conceive and effect them, required most of all the resolu-

tion, the carelessness of consequences, that would persuade men
to do what needed doing regardless of convention, custom, or
law.

Already, respect for law was wavering. The Guardians had
seized Ricketts' circus with no legal warrant. The Mayor himself had done arbitrary things, and committed the council to
expenditures beyond the budget, far beyond his powers. This
he had done willingly, but certainly not with the unhesitating
confidence of settled and sure legal authorization.

The state constitution of 1790, and the city charter, had
not been framed to care for a crisis like this. A firm, strong
hand was needed, a hand that would grasp authority wherever
it lay and rule with such force as could be exerted. As in
1776, so now the city had to be governed, in defect of properly
constituted authority, by those who cared. Mayor Clarkson
was aware of the misery in Ricketts' circus, and of the determination of the neighboring householders to wipe it out, by
fire if necessary. Mayor Clarkson was one of those who cared.
On Thursday, August 29, after receiving the Governor's letter,
he called the Guardians together—seven of the fourteen showed
up—and such of the aldermen as he could find. A general
discussion of the epidemic was held. Most of all that lazaretto
was needed, that "hospital in an airy and healthy place" the
College of Physicians had urged. So far, no one had offered
his country home, and time could not be lost in dickering for
a purchase. The assembled magistrates determined simply to
take whatever place they could find.

Encouraged by the Mayor the Guardians resolved, even as
Clarkson was writing his reply to the Governor that Thursday
evening, to "use their utmost exertion to procure a suitable
house," out of town but as close as was safe, for the reception
of the stricken poor. They would engage physicians, nurses,
attendants, purchase all necessary supplies, appoint inspectors
in each district of the city to investigate cases, administer relief,
and if required remove the poor to the new hospital. They
would appoint a physician and—how welcome Clarkson's firm-

ness must have been—they would draw upon the Mayor for such money as they needed.

Money could stop the plague. The Governor had committed the legislature, the Mayor could now commit the Governor, the Guardians could go the limit. They did, and their search was quickly finished. On high ground at the northwest edge of the city stood a huge mansion, a famous old place known to every Philadelphian. Providentially, it was empty. The Guardians could scarcely have made another choice, yet they proceeded with some reluctance. This was one of Philadelphia's most famous and respected homes.

Nearly seventy years before, the great lawyer, Andrew Hamilton, architect of Independence Hall, had purchased from Mrs. William Penn about 150 acres of Springettsbury Manor, lying along the city's northern boundary. His lands, extending between Twelfth and Nineteenth streets north of Vine, adjoining another parcel he owned within the city, gave Hamilton a farm half as large as the corporate limits of Philadelphia itself. Atop the highest rise on his farm, Hamilton built about 1740 a noble residence with numerous outbuildings, giving his home the name "Bush Hill." He did not enjoy his splendor very long, for next year he died and was buried at Bush Hill. He bequeathed the estate to his son James.

James, for many years Deputy Governor of the province, was an old bachelor when the Revolution came. He remained loyal, and followed the British to New York, where he died toward the end of the war. Bush Hill passed to his nephew William, but William had been for some time living in England, and the great house continued to stand empty, a conspicuous relic of past grandeur. In 1788 the elaborate federal pageant on the Fourth of July had ended at Union Green, in front of Bush Hill, where seventeen thousand people gathered. When the new federal government moved to the city in 1790, Vice-President John Adams occupied the mansion for two years; now in 1793 it was vacant again.

Abigail Adams had thought the house beautiful, the interior

workmanship particularly fine. The British back in '77 had robbed it of its principal glory by cutting down all the trees in front of the mansion "and leaving it wholly Naked," but behind was a fine grove with gravel walks. Eight months of the year it was a "delicious" place, two and a half miles from town; only the bad roads in winter gave Mrs. Adams cause to complain.

The Guardians had no doubt Bush Hill would be the best location for their hospital, but they hesitated to seize the property of an absent gentleman. They decided to leave the mansion alone and take one of the outbuildings, for which purpose, securing the prior assent of the Governor, eight Guardians with Alderman Hilary Baker rode out to Bush Hill on Saturday, August 31. The tenant, Thomas Boyles, who with his wife and six children occupied the outbuilding, met this deputation with a firm resolve to defeat whatever claim of law might be supporting them. He positively refused to give up his home. The Guardians were equally resolved, however. They wasted no time in fruitless argument with the tenant, but left him and seized the mansion house itself.

It was a bold step, one bound to cause serious problems. Hamilton, when he learned his property had been taken without his knowledge or consent, averred he had "been hardly treated on the occasion." But the Guardians were in no mood to think of legal problems. They occupied, as it was later described,

all that part of Bush Hill within the circular Ha Ha on the South, bounded by a line extending from the western end of the said Ha Ha to South East of the Grave-yard, thence by a line to the new ditch, which encloses the pine grove on the North, thence by the several courses of the said ditch round the grove to the North East corner of the old green-house foundation, thence along the Northern side of the coach-house and stables and the Eastern side of the same to the gate on Callowhill street, with the use of the lane to the East end of the Ha Ha wall, with the Mansion-house, Kitchen, stables etc.

Bush Hill became in this manner the hospital in an "airy and healthy place." To it on the evening of Saturday, August 31, the

Guardians removed the four paupers at the circus still living, the first of a grim train that in the next fortnight would turn the handsome old mansion itself into a dread charnel house of fear, dismal suffering, and death.

Philadelphia had endured twelve days of the plague—twelve days since Rush had seen Cathy LeMaigre, and confounded the citizens with his news. In twelve days the city had fallen apart. What had to be done, Mayor Clarkson had seen to, but in the thirty-one days of August an enormous number of Philadelphians had died. The Mayor cautiously estimated 140, Dr. Rush said 325. Perhaps both were wrong, but figures meant little, now or later: now, because the fever struck with such horrid randomness; later, because September was to be so immeasurably worse.

Crisis

Observation without principles is nothing but empiricism. . . . It is by means of principles in medicine that a physician can practise with safety to his patients, and satisfaction to himself.
—BENJAMIN RUSH

ON Sunday, September 1, Thomas Jefferson sat writing letters on the terrace of the country home he rented out near Gray's Ferry on the Schuylkill's bank. It was a pleasant place, airy and light, with fine old trees. Across the river were the amazing gardens of the botanists John and William Bartram, where the Secretary of State occasionally went for a stroll. During the summer heat he wrote, received, and dined on his terrace in the open air. Frequently his friend Dr. Hutchinson would dine with him, discuss Genêt and his schemes, the whole question of neutrality, or Jefferson's resignation and imminent retirement, for the Secretary was winding up his affairs and preparing for a final holiday.

To James Madison in Virginia, Jefferson wrote that Sunday of the fever. Everyone who could was fleeing, he told Madison, and he feared that the panic of country people would add famine to disease in the afflicted city. He had instructed his daughter Maria to stay out at Gray's Ferry, but he himself had to go to town every day. Jefferson watched the fever closely. At first, three out of every four stricken had died; even now one out of three was lost. Death came between the second and eighth day.

A week later, the Secretary wrote again to Madison. Daily

deaths had increased, he estimated, to eleven. About thirty-three new cases were reported every twenty-four hours, and around 330 patients were being treated. The physicians saw no way of stopping it. "They agree it is a nondescript disease, and no two agree in any one part of their process of cure." On September 11, Jefferson told another correspondent that deaths would pass two hundred for the week, and he dreaded the fever's spread to other towns.

Actually, Jefferson was low in his figures. Sunday the first of September passed, and seventeen had died. Monday the second took eighteen more, Tuesday eleven, Wednesday twenty-three, so the incredible rolls read. More than twenty burials each day the rest of the week were recorded. Then on Sunday, September 8, came a ghastly total of forty-two. Monday the ninth and Tuesday the tenth the figure hovered at thirty, but by Friday it had reached thirty-seven, and on Saturday the 14th, forty-eight.

The exodus continued, more houses were closed, people sickened of the fever, and they sickened of fear. Panic spread from heart to heart, fear paralyzed the whole as spasms racked the stricken, panic was the vicious ally of disease.

A cheerful countenance was nowhere to be seen. Dr. Rush met only tears and silent grief; once the happy smile of a two-year-old child brought him up short in shocked surprise. Funerals now were conducted as the College had urged, in lonely haste. "It is indeed truly affecting to see a solitary corpse," Rush wrote his wife on Sunday the first, "on the shafts and wheels of a chair, conducted thro' our streets without a single attendant in some cases, and with only 8 or 10 in any instance, and they at a small distance from it on the foot pavement."

The only persons in the streets were physicians or those looking for physicians, nurses, bleeders, or servants of the dead. Yet Rush realized with horror that September first was only the beginning of the pestilence. It was an appalling thought.

The Doctor reflected on those he had lost. "I can truly say I am more anxious to be pardoned, and to be delivered from the guilt, dominion and punishment of my sins, than to be preserved from the present pestilential fever," he confessed to Julia. "If I survive the present dangers to which I am exposed, what offering of gratitude will ever equal the infinite weight of my obligations to my gracious deliverer? You must help me to be more humble, more patient, more devout, and more self-denied in everything."

It was a mood strange to Rush, this praying for humility and patience—stranger particularly in view of the great discovery he was to make before September was many hours older. By the end of this week his confidence would be restored, but on September first he was as confused, as alarmed, as apprehensive as all the other doctors. On the fourth, he scratched a hurried note to his anxious wife:

I am now waiting with great anxiety for my breakfast, having had a call from my bed. I was much too fatigued to fill my paper last night, and too much hurried this morning. I lose not a moment. The bed my kind sister provided for me in the back room lies unoccupied all day. Adieu. Love to all. "Brethren pray for us." Hark! a knock at the door! Alas, it is called to Mrs. Boggs at Bishop White. Again adieu. The delay of a minute seems a year to a patient after a physician is sent for.

Others besides Dr. Rush were praying for guidance also, and many supplemented their prayers by applying to the famous physician for leadership. Samuel Powel, Speaker of the Senate, had spent an uneasy Saturday, for he feared, indeed he knew, the legislature would be restless when it met again after the week-end recess. From his elegant house in Third Street on the evening of Sunday the first, Powel despatched a servant round the corner with a note to Rush. The Speaker would be obliged if Dr. Rush would inform him please if the putrid disorder was abating or increasing? "The Apprehensions of many of the Members [of the Assembly] are great," Powel wrote, "& if you can enable me to allay them, the public Business will probably proceed, but should the Case unfortunately prove otherwise I believe that it will be impracticable to keep the Members in Town."

Dr. Rush read the note, turned it over, and wrote on the back a brief message: "I know of but one certain preventative of the disorder, & that is to keep at a distance from infected persons and places."

Mr. Powel had his answer. But he also had his colleagues. On Monday, when the Assembly met, committees were appointed by each house to report upon the expediency of adjourning. The committees conferred, but on Tuesday had to report disagreement. The Senate on Tuesday therefore acted independently, and passed a resolution, "that the Legislature will rise tomorrow," and sent it to the House for concurrence.

The House was reluctant. There was much business to do, not the least important item of which was the impeachment of John Nicholson, the Comptroller, which the House had brought and the Senate ought to try. On Wednesday, September 4, instead of concurring in adjournment, the representatives asked the senators please to set a time for the trial. The senators considered; Anthony Morris moved that since so many members were sick or absent, and all were alarmed, the present session was no fit time to try an impeachment. This motion was voted down, so the Senate decided, if it had to conduct the trial, to get on with it at once. The sergeant at arms was sent out to serve a summons on John Nicholson.

Comptroller Nicholson, however, was nowhere to be found. The sergeant at arms came back with his subpoena not served, so Morris once again made his motion to drop the impeachment for the present session, and the motion this time carried. Thereupon the House sent in two additional charges against Nicholson, and after a busy afternoon of routine work the legislators went home for the night—not, however, before they heard (and rejected) a motion from a Quaker member to close the theatres and places of amusement in the city on account of the plague, and to enjoin the people to humble themselves before Almighty God.

Thursday the fifth, fewer members showed up. The day began with an unexpected message from the Governor: the fever was

raging, said Mifflin, yet ships were still coming in from the
West Indies without inspection. And from elsewhere, too—
at that very moment a vessel from Ireland with a large number
of feverish aboard lay at Mud Island—it was the *Hope* out of
Londonderry—yet the law concerning the health office was still
"exceedingly defective" and no funds had been granted to support and attend the sick at the quarantine station. Would not
the legislature act immediately, as the Governor had asked?

Both houses responded at once. Someone unearthed the old
quarantine act, copied most of it, and introduced it as a bill "to
prevent infectious diseases being brought into the province"—
so hurried were the members that they forgot to change the
old word "province" to "commonwealth." It was rushed
through, sent to Mifflin for signature, received back, and en-
rolled immediately. It granted special emergency powers to the
Governor for the duration of the pestilence. Then Senator Morris for the third time moved "that the Legislature will rise this
day." The representatives hesitated no longer. Both houses settled their accounts, and without further delay adjourned till
December.

"The members," Representative Jacob Hiltzheimer wrote in
his diary, "decline remaining in the city." He himself returned
to his home at Seventh and the High to care for his family.
Senator Anthony Morris went out to his little summer home
on the banks of the Schuylkill, where he found crowded into
the flimsy lodge his wife, two daughters, a cousin with his wife
and daughter, three of Dr. Thomas Parke's children, a nurse,
and servants from three or four of the city's greatest families.

Governor Mifflin, committed to the import-quarantine theory and now left in complete charge by the legislature, took
other steps under the new law. He directed Mayor Clarkson to
prevent any person off the ship *Hope* from entering the city.
He ordered Nathaniel Falconer, Health Officer of the Port, to
prevent any vessel from the West Indies coming further up the
river than Mud Island until it had been examined; and to de-
tain any vessel from anywhere with sick people aboard until

the Physician of the Port had inspected it. Further, he directed Falconer to do everything and anything necessary to relieve the public from the calamity, attend the patients at Bush Hill, hire two assistants at $3 per day, engage a boat with oarsmen to speed his inspection of vessels.

Then the Governor left town. He was said to be ill himself; he went out to his country place at Falls of Schuylkill, where the air was clean and fresh.

Perhaps he felt like Rush's neighbor, attorney William Lewis, who had fled with his family on August 27 and wrote Dr. Rush from the country:

A large City with the Houses shut up & the Streets empty except the french Sailors, People of St. Domingo of all Colours with their Heads tied a few Citizens whom you do not know posting along with Sponges in their noses & the Herse Constantly passing exhibits such a melancholly picture that I never left Philad^a. with so much pleasure as yesterday nor never found Such Pleasure in the Country as I do today . . .

II

Mayor Clarkson had no intention of leaving town. In these first two weeks of September he saw one alderman after another go off; frequently only he and John Barclay would meet— devoted Barclay, his predecessor as mayor, now president of the Bank of Pennsylvania, who resolved to stay at his double post even after the fever struck his daughter, then him. Of the Guardians of the Poor for the city only three remained by the end of the first week in September: James Wilson, Jacob Tomkins, Jr., William Sansom.

The Mayor could actually do little for the time being, but he set an example of courage and firmness. Every day he could be seen riding down Second Street to City Hall, where he sat hour after hour in his chambers, poring over papers, meeting problems that had no solution, peering with his odd gaze at his visitors. The Guardians, old Barclay, Dr. Rush, officers of state and national governments all sent to him for news, advice, or help. He could do nothing—not even when he heard the Governor had left, or when young James Wilson, the Guardian, brought him news of conditions at Bush Hill.

Of course, things were bad there. To seize a long-closed house, move patients in the same day, provide no nurses or attendants, was bound to cause trouble. And, of course, none but the most desperate characters could be induced to serve there. Clarkson told people of the need, he asked for help, he conferred with the doctors. He appointed Physick, Cathrall, Annan, and Leib—young men—to go each day to visit the sick. And Dr. Rush sent him another young chap, Charles Caldwell, a second-year medical student from North Carolina. Caldwell explained to Rush that the family he lived with had fled the city. He moved in with a second family, and they likewise left. Did Dr. Rush know anywhere he could live? Rush told him of the hospital just opened at Bush Hill, where qualified pupils were needed as resident aids to prepare and administer prescriptions, superintend nurses, and do whatever else seemed necessary. No pay was given, but it would be a splendid opportunity to see the fever.

Caldwell set out at once, and within an hour was engaged on "melancholy and momentous duties." He found everything "limited, crude and insufficient," the nurses few and inexperienced. "In fact, the whole establishment being, in its character as a hospital, the product of but two or three days' labor, by men altogether unversed in such business, was a likeness in miniature of the city at the time, a scene of deep confusion and distress, not to say of utter desolation."

Confusion, distress, desolation—that was the picture Clarkson confronted. He, like all the others, was a man unversed in such business. He tried to find people to assist the Guardians in the city and at Bush Hill, but it was hopeless. Young Caldwell was the only recruit.

He could, however, use the newspapers. The Mayor had the clean-up ordinances printed and reprinted, and he used such resources as he had. They were slender enough. Not to him, but to Mifflin, had the legislature granted emergency powers, and Mifflin had left. Nathaniel Falconer proceeded with the steps the Governor had ordered, but certain of the passengers from the *Hope* out of Londonderry wandered away from their internment at State Island, so the Mayor ordered them rounded up. Yet he had no magistrates or constables to order, and for want of better means used Brown's paper to call upon "all good citizens" for the purpose. The "good citizens" showed no interest in apprehending passengers from the *Hope*. Demoralization was too far advanced. A doctor even noted that bodies of several victims lay unburied in the Potter's Field.

The Port Physician, Dr. Hutchinson, by the end of August was desperately ill, and this first week in September was hovering on the edge of death. He arranged with young Dr. Mease to take all his charity patients. If Hutchinson recovered, a permanent partnership was to be formed. Meanwhile, vessels came in with no medical inspection.

Back into the papers came the old recommendation to destroy the plague by heavy smoke, though no one did anything about it. And though the cannon was silent, the popular practice of purifying the air by firing off guns, which the Mayor and Governor had encouraged, continued both indoors and outdoors. Houses rocked with explosions of muskets, and smoked with the acrid fumes of gunpowder deflagrated on charcoal. But outdoors the practice was "accompanied with damage and inconvenience." It became unsafe to walk in the streets because of earnest citizens' firing their muskets, so Clarkson ordered the shooting stopped. He took the step the more willingly, he said, since the practice was "considered by the Physicians as highly injurious."

The doctors had no rest. They were called to dozens of patients daily, and their waiting rooms were filled when they got home. "Continue to commit me by your prayers to the protection of that Being who has so often manifested his goodness to our family by the preservation of my life," Rush begged his wife. He had no will of his own, but placed himself in God's hands. "I even strive to subdue my sympathy for my patients, otherwise I should sink under the accumulated load of misery I am obliged to contemplate," he wrote.

Other doctors were sinking under the fever itself. Rush watched with great care the illness of Hutchinson; by September 3 Kuhn, M'Ilvaine, Carson, and Wistar had all taken the disease. Carson and Kuhn improved slowly, M'Ilvaine recovered, and Wistar, watched over by his devoted pupil Billy Bache, seemed to be safe. Doctors were keenly aware of their danger.

Yet there was time for public controversy. In *Dunlap's Daily Advertiser* on September 2 appeared an attack on Rush's theory about the coffee, signed "Medicus." Rush had published a description of the fever, attributing it to local filth. "Medicus," a contagionist following Cullen's nosology, remarked that the damaged coffee had "made as much noise, and with equal cause, as the scratchings of the Cock Lane Ghost." He told of some poor people from down on Passyunk Road (below Gray's Ferry) who had gathered up some of the coffee from Ball's Wharf, taken it home and brewed it, yet remained in perfect health. Obviously, "Medicus" argued, there could be no noxious exhalation from it.

This article, of course, offended Rush, but it caused acute unhappiness of another kind to Dr. Benjamin Duffield, who had casually mentioned to Rush in conversation that he doubted if the coffee was the cause of the contagion. Duffield had not written the "Medicus" article, but he knew Rush would think he had. He sent his distinguished colleague a letter denying the authorship and repudiating all "such illiberal anonymous Slanderers." To Duffield's surprise, Rush answered cryptically, charging that Duffield's criticism had injured him in the city. The chagrined Duffield responded that he was entirely unconscious of having criticized or injured his friend. "If to differ from you in medical Opinions is a Crime," he told Rush, "it is one that every man must at one Time or other of his Life, be guilty of with some of his Fellow Travellers in the Difficult Road of Science."

Such differences in medical opinion, crimes or not, were becoming serious public matters. Already, in the varying techniques of treatment, the doctors were discovering profound and disturbing antagonisms, which would produce theoretical conflicts that almost slipped American medical science from her moorings.

As every doctor realized by the first week in September, traditional means of coping with the disease were hopelessly ineffectual. No one found anything that worked. John Thompson Young, who practiced in Pine Street, had seen his first case on August 1. For seven days he prescribed evacuants, and as the patient grew worse he blistered him on the wrists and back of the neck. These blisters failed to heal, but discharged "an acrid offensive fluid" until death.

Dr. Cathrall had early decided to proceed by three steps in his cases in Water Street: first, he would reduce inflammatory action; second, he would alleviate symptoms, and third, support the tone and vigor of the system. He began in August by bleeding and purging, but soon gave up bleeding. Later at Bush Hill he would resume this practice, after Physick's autopsies and his own had shown stomachs inflamed and the organs full of "redundant fluid blood."

Dr. Adam Kuhn before he fell ill had seen a number of cases of fever. Kuhn, a careful observer and more original in theory than most, refused to be dominated by any general hypotheses. Only seven out of his sixty-odd cases had really been yellow fever, he averred; the rest were merely the annual remittent and intermittent autumnal disorder. For the yellow fever he had a cure, and he claimed extraordinary success. The first thing was to remove debility and putrefaction, not to reduce inflammation. Therefore he gave no purge, unless a mild one for costiveness. Nausea he relieved by camomile tea and, if it continued, by effervescing salts, vitriol, the bark or laudanum, or all in carefully contrived combination, and a plaster applied to the pit of the stomach. If the patient could not retain the bark when taken orally, he injected a clyster of water, laudanum, Madeira wine, and the bark in powdered form every four hours.

Wines and lemonade were to be given at first, the debility overcome by a regimen of ripe fruits, sago with wine, and rich wines. But, Dr. Kuhn added, "I place the greatest dependence for the cure of the disease, on throwing cool water twice a day over the naked body." To do this he placed the patient in a large empty tub and poured on him a couple of buckets of water 70 to 80 degrees Fahrenheit. Then he wiped him dry and put him to bed. This, he insisted, always resulted in "great refreshment to the patient."

Except for the cold baths, this system of Kuhn was a mild one. It was really a system of letting nature do the work. Dr. Edward Stevens, "eminent and worthy physician from St. Croix, who happened to be in our city," followed the same method. He was particularly opposed to evacuations or bleeding. The disease was, Stevens agreed with Kuhn, more a putrid fever than an inflammatory one, and ought to be treated by strengthening the system, not weakening an inflammation. Actually, such a cure by cordial, tonic remedies, and cool baths had been described fourteen years earlier by a West India physician in a letter to Dr. Lettsom of London, and Lettsom had given it currency. But Dr. George Logan of Stenton pointed out that it had never worked, even in the islands where it originated. There, evacuations were always used at the outset of the fever, and the mild remedy was completely useless. As Logan saw it, there were two needs: first, remove congestions in the abdominal vessels; and second, remove the atonia of the extreme vessels, and promote perspiration. The methods of doing so were bleeding and purging.

Other doctors favored "a union of the evacuating and tonic remedies"—evacuating, to reduce inflammation; tonic, to overcome putrescence. The French physicians and Santo Domingans had their own technique: "nitre and cremor tartar, in small doses, century tea, camphor, and several other warm medicines; subacid drinks [like lemon or lime juice] taken in large quantities, the warm bath, and moderate bleedings."

None of these remedies worked. Especially, the American doctors thought, the French cure failed. Dr. John Penington of Sassafras Street declared he had lost six patients by the French method, and Dr. Robert Johnson of the Dispensary told Rush "with great concern, about two weeks before he died, that he had not recovered a single patient by them."

Rush tried all cures. He had begun in August with gentle purges and mild bleedings "to abstract excess of stimulus from the system," and recommended cool air, cold drinks, low diet, and cold baths. This had resulted in nothing at all, and on that August 19 when he emerged from Cathy LeMaigre's house with his discovery of the true nature of the disease, he changed his method. He administered "a gentle vomit of ipecacuanha" on the first day of fever, following it with "the usual remedies for exciting the action of the sanguiferous system." When these failed he began to experiment desperately.

I gave bark in all its usual forms of infusion, powder and tincture. I joined wine, brandy, and aromatics with it. I applied blisters to the limbs, neck and head. Finding them all ineffectual, I attempted to rouse the system by wrapping the whole body, agreeably to Dr. Hume's practice in blankets dipped in warm vinegar. To these remedies I added one more: I rubbed the right side with mercurial ointment, with a view of exciting the action of the vessels in the whole system through the medium of the liver . . .

None of these practices achieved anything. Yet Rush refused to believe the disease could not be cured. He went to ask advice of Dr. Stevens. Edward Stevens' firmness of manner, prominent political connections, and West India origin gave him the air of authority. Stevens "politely" informed Rush that he had long ago abandoned purges in yellow fever, and used only the mild remedies: the bark in large quantities as a clyster and in other doses, wine and a cold bath, in short, Lettsom's cure.

This sounded reasonable to Rush, for his books taught that when the bowels were full of vicious humors produced by faulty circulation, the bark "by bracing the solids" enabled them "to throw off the excrementitious fluids, by the proper emunctories." Accordingly, for a while he followed the method of Stevens and Kuhn, even to the buckets full of cold water thrown on the patients frequently, but after a few days he gave all this up, concluding Stevens was no more right than anyone else.

Inexorably the deaths increased. Charles Biddle was reminded of Benjamin Franklin's observation that in Barbados the inhabitants began to recover from the fever only after the doctors had run out of medicine. And Stephen Girard, in the midst of his mercantile activities, inveighed bitterly against the stupidity of "our Esculapians." Rush was frantic. "Heaven alone bore witness to the anguish of my soul in this awful situation," he wrote. Yet he did not give up hope. Convinced that Divine Providence had not failed to provide a cure for every illness, he applied himself "with fresh ardour to the investigation of the disease before me." His method of investigating was to turn to his books. He ransacked his library, searching his great authors for descriptions of yellow fever, only to find their accounts of symptoms and cures foolishly contradictory, altogether inapplicable.

The great authors, that is, were contradictory and inapplicable. There was a lesser author who was not. Poring over his books, Rush recalled an old manuscript he had. Dr. Franklin had given it to him. It was John Mitchell's description of the yellow fever in Virginia in 1741, which the physician and map maker had sent to Franklin many years before. Rush remembered having made use of it in preparing lectures at the University. Now he went back to read it again. Page after page of the largest size double folio Rush turned over, for Mitchell's essay was no trivial performance. It was strikingly original, and Rush found himself reading with keen attention. Suddenly there leaped from the page Mitchell's observation that in yellow fever the abdominal viscera were filled with blood, and must be cleaned out by immediate evacuation. Thus "the very minera of the disease, proceeding from the putrid miasmata fermenting with the salivary, bilious, and other inquiline humours of the body, is sometimes eradicated by timely emptying the abdominal viscera, on which it first fixes. . . ." Afterwards a gentle sweat would follow, and continue to purge the body of the vicious humors.

When the stomach was full of offensive matter, Mitchell declared, or inflamed, contracted, and convulsed, no laudable sweat could be procured. Such matter had to be removed. To remove it, nature would have to be assisted, even superseded, by the physician's art. This was always true in acute putrid fevers.

"An *ill-timed scrupulousness about the weakness of the body*" on the part of a physician was fatal, Rush read. It was that very weakness which made evacuations necessary, and rendered nature unable to achieve them. The physician should produce these evacuations by *"lenitive chologoque purges."* Mitchell asserted boldly, "I have given a purge . . . when *the pulse has been so low, that it could hardly be felt,* and the *debility extreme,* yet *both one and the other* have been *restored by it."*

"Here I paused," Rush wrote later. "A new train of ideas suddenly broke in upon my mind." It was extraordinary doctrine. Doctors had ever regarded their efforts as merely assistant to nature, yet Mitchell was blandly proclaiming the physician must domineer over nature, scorn her, command her, anticipate her, ignore her. Rush's imagination was immediately inflamed. He, like all other doctors, had set out to strengthen, not weaken; to restore, not tear down; yet he had lost patients. Could it be that weakness should be made weaker, after Mitchell's fashion? Purges so far had failed, and so had bleeding. Stevens, Kuhn, and the others had rejected them both. But Rush, absorbed with Mitchell's manuscript, received its doctrine as revelation. "Dr. Mitchell in a moment dissipated my ignorance and fears. . . ." He realized that the trouble had been, not that he purged, but that he purged too gently. He must overcome his "ill-timed scrupulousness about the weakness of the body." He must boldly empty the abdominal viscera. He must purge with a mighty effect.

Years before, he recalled, he and the late Dr. Clarkson (the Mayor's brother) had consulted together over a case of bilious pleurisy. He had prescribed bleeding, Clarkson purgation. When the patient recovered, Clarkson remarked, "Doctor, you and I have each a great fault in our practice; I do not bleed enough, you do not purge enough."

Now the strongest purge Rush had ever seen was Dr. Thomas Young's "Ten-and-Ten" in the Revolutionary army—ten grains of calomel (mercury) and ten of jalap. This Rush resolved to use. But it was an enormous dose, far stronger than medical men thought safe. Soldiers in the field were sturdy and strong, but citizens at home, weakened by the heats of the summer, softly conditioned by a peaceful life—were they fit subjects for the great Ten-and-Ten? How could Rush dare experiment thus with human life?

It was told around the city how Rush first dared. One day (August 29) in his rounds he found a man all alone in a closed house, deserted by his family, obviously at the very point of death. If Rush did nothing the man would surely die, and whatever he tried probably would not save him. No witnesses were present, no weeping family, no consulting physicians or observing students. Rush forced down the dying man's throat "a medicine which had for some days been upon his mind"— the mercury and jalap. He stayed by the patient "till the operation was over." Amazingly, the purge worked, and still more amazingly, the man at once showed signs of recovery.

The Doctor controlled his excitement. He wrote Julia calmly that he had tried his new medicine, "I think with some advantage." He began to use it in other cases, and to experiment. The jalap he increased to fifteen grains, to speed the operation. Still it was too slow, so he developed a regimen of three doses of ten and fifteen, one every six hours, until they produced four or five large evacuations.

This was the amazing remedy Dr. Rush discovered among

his books, the remedy Kuhn would call "a murderous dose," Dr. Barton "a devil of a dose," Dr. Hodge "a dose for a horse."

With the purge to draw off putrid and excess matter, Rush further combined the "antiphlogiston" regimen—cold drinks, cool air, cold baths, soft diet, and bloodletting—to "abstract excess of stimulus from the system." Bloodletting he had generally tried, but in small amounts. Now he realized he must take enough blood to remove all inflammatory stimulus—to reduce all stimulus, indeed, that might operate on the "inquiline humours" of the body.

This new system seemed to work. Indeed, it far exceeded Rush's expectations. It "perfectly cured" four out of five patients, he declared. Even Richard Spain, a blockmaker, who had been given up for lost after lying twelve hours without a pulse, recovered from dosages of 80 grains of calomel and 120 grains of rhubarb and jalap. Lawyer Lewis, Dr. M'Ilvaine, Mrs. Bethal, her two sons and a serving maid, and nine members of Peter Baynton's family were "trophies of the new cure."

Rush was delighted with his startling method. He no longer concealed his excitement. By September 2 he began stopping other physicians in the streets and telling them about it. When Dr. Wistar fell ill, at Rush's advice he took the great purge. Wistar was not fully convinced, but he did improve. And to Dr. Hutchinson's bedside Rush went, to recover the dying Port Physician with mercury and jalap. Hutchinson indignantly refused the strange medicine. Young Barton, his physician, coldly informed Rush that it would be curious to prescribe a purge, since Dr. Hutchinson had passed "near thirty stools in three days." But Rush put this down to the animosity Hutchinson had always entertained for him, and went on his enthusiastic way. On September 3 he informed the Fellows of the College of his cure, and boldly he wrote to Julia that he recovered eight out of twelve patients with one day's treatment. On the fourth, he declared that nine out of ten who took his purge immediately on their first attack recovered. On the fifth he wrote that though the pestilence spread, it was no more fatal than a common bilious fever when treated with his mercury compound. "I now save 29 out of 30 of all to whom I am called on the first day and many to whom I am called after it."

He even believed his great purge and copious bloodletting could prevent as well as cure the disease. "I owe these discoveries, as well as my preservation, to the prayers of my friends," he wrote.

No more would Rush pray for humility, self-denial, and patience. He had found the cure.

Never before did I experience such sublime joy as I now felt in contemplating the success of my remedies. It repaid me for all the toils and studies of my life. The conquest of this formidable disease was not the effect of accident, nor of the application of a single remedy; but it was the triumph of a principle in medicine.

A new principle in medicine was what many had been waiting for. Samuel Powel Griffitts, gentle Quaker though he was, adopted the great purge at once, and Rush immediately became his fast friend. "We consult together every day," he wrote. Dr. Say found the new theory the perfect answer he had been seeking. Dr. Penington ran across Third Street in a transport to tell Rush that the disease yielded in every case to mercury and jalap.

The prostrate Wistar, enduring Rush's enthusiasm as well as his medicines, smiled when the Doctor mentioned the dangers of the plague. "You cannot die now, Dr.," Wistar remarked. "The pleasure of your discovery must like a cordial keep you alive." This Rush admitted, confessing it had "infused a vigor into my body and mind, which has contributed very much to support me under my present exertions." Former students, Woodhouse, Mease, Annan, Porter, Leib, at once rallied to their master's strange pennon; but there, for the moment, recruitment stopped.

As the deaths mounted, Rush in person, in public writings, in private letters, proclaimed his great principle. All his confidence flowed back, all his restraints were thrown off. He could only wonder why others refused to accept his truth.

III

Others did refuse. Dr. Rush's truth was much too startling for them. Physicians realized he was approaching the realms of God's natural order, and approaching with violence; laymen realized their simple cures were not without effect. The household remedies continued to be advertised and hawked about. Jesuits' Bark was described in the papers, and a correspondent in Brown's *Federal Gazette* praised Delaney's Aromatic Distilled Vinegar as the only sovereign remedy against "the prevailing fatal epidemic." Another (more helpful than he knew) pointed out that fresh pennyroyal laid on the pillow would keep away mosquitoes, and asked, since it was so powerful why might it not be a good preventive against the infectious disorder? To "Quaestor Veritatis," who had denied the disease was yellow fever, "Aroteus, Jun." (Charles Caldwell) replied with heat proving the epidemic "nothing else than the genuine Typhus of Dr. Cullen; the jail-fever of Pringle—the hospital fever of Lind, and the ship fever of Blane, which are all so many different names for the same malady." The causes were confined air, crowded apartments, the "defect of cleanliness and putrifying animal and vegetable substances."

Young Charles Caldwell, even under classical pseudonyms, carried no weight in the city, but he must have pleased Rush by this defense, for the previous spring he had opposed, both in newspaper articles and in the lecture hall, this very doctrine of the unity of fevers which Rush enthusiastically expounded. Caldwell believed himself now convinced by a fact, not a theory.

Dr. Joseph Goss of Second Street averred that he had treated above sixty patients with considerable success by inducing a heavy sweat for twelve hours, giving ditiny tea with molasses and a decoction of twelve turnips, one endive, and eight carrots boiled in a gallon of water down to three quarts, a clyster every four or five hours, balsam or camphor for coughing, and ipecacuanha for nausea.

"I. W." replied to this, accusing Dr. Goss of ignorance, charlatanry, and quackery, urging victims to go to men of education and experience—a strange way to use an established practitioner like Goss. Less worldly writers deemed the fever caused by the pride and corruption of the citizens, their playhouses, circus, palaces, carriages, and costly edifices; they commended prayer and submission to God in place of flight or medicine.

Meanwhile, among the doctors several were taking specific attitudes on Rush's cure. Not only Hutchinson refused mercury purges and bleedings; Kuhn likewise advised everyone to reject them. A greater mind than either of these was addressing the problem, however: Dr. William Currie, working as feverishly as Rush during the days, spent his nights composing a pamphlet on his own methods of prevention and cure. On September 4 Currie delivered his manuscript to Thomas Dobson in Second Street. Dobson put his printers to work at once. In two days he had set up and issued a pamphlet of thirty-six pages: *A Description of the Malignant, Infectious Fever Prevailing at Present in Philadelphia; with an Account of the Means to Prevent Infection, and the Remedies and Method of Treatment, Which Have Been Found Most Successful. By William Currie, Fellow of the College of Physicians.* This was the first book on the fever, the first of many; it was the first authentic handbook people had.

Currie described the symptoms of the fever in language so simple that laymen could easily understand and recognize them. Then he stated, with no qualification, that the infection was produced by specific bodily contagion, and might be "communicated from those labouring under the disease, to persons in the most perfect state of health."

It was communicable only under certain circumstances, however, and only directly by the people infected, or by clothes and porous substances which had been in contact with the sick. It certainly was not carried by the air. "Burning heaps of odorous and noisom substances in the streets is therefore not only useless, but injurious, as it not only consumes or changes the quality of the pure or vital air of the atmosphere, but conveys into it from the burning materials, a proportionable quantity of deleterious gas, commonly called fixed air." People walking in the streets encountered no danger; only those did who were confined in the same room with victims, or came in contact with the body or bedclothes of a patient or nurse, or received "the breath, or the scent of the several excretions of the sick." Cleanliness, ventilation, moderate exercise, sensible diet, and temperance would protect every individual, and the whole city.

All the familiar nostrums—the tarred rope, camphor bags, amulets of dried frogs, vinegar sponges, segars—Currie denounced as more evil than good, particularly because they made people think about the fever and were depressing. The best and only neutralizer of contagion was, he asserted, "the pure vital air of the atmosphere." Vital air was what made fires burn, and people breathe. "This salubrious aeriform fluid may therefore be most usefully employed for restoring to health the unfortunate sufferers. . . ." Nitre should be frequently deflagrated on burning charcoal in sickrooms, for this produced an abundance of vital air. Other ways of manufacturing the salubrious aeriform fluid were to pour vinegar on a hot iron, build fires in chimneys, put about the room growing plants or vessels of cottonseed water on which peppergrass was sown, for the grass would immediately vegetate and purify the air (though the vessel should be removed every night).

Currie described his method of cure, far different from Rush's new discovery, from Kuhn's system, or Cathrall's: tartar emetic in tea or barley water every half-hour until effective, next day a mild purgative, sudorific anodyne at night, salt of tartar in lime juice given in barley water or gruel every two hours to encourage perspiration, or laudanum and ammonia for the same purpose; he recommended bathing the feet and hands in vinegar and water; soaking the bed linen in vinegar, drying thoroughly, changing twice daily. The patient should lie in the middle of the room with no curtains and all the air possible. "Perhaps lying in a tent placed in a dry verdant field would be preferable to the most spacious chamber."

Currie rejected bleeding. He observed that "the activity of the pulse and heat of the skin in its first stage, certainly call for the antiphlogistic regimen, and such medicines as abate arterial action," but he further noted that "a state of debility very soon and constantly follows this state of increased action and apparent power in the arterial system," and accordingly decided bloodletting was too strong a measure.

He also rejected mercury. Mild purging diminished arterial tension slowly and safely, without contributing to debility, so he used only mild purges—if calomel, a very small amount, with or without laudanum. He favored blisters between the shoulders and on each leg; wine, bark, a cataplasm of mustard and vinegar, peppermint, elixir of vitriol, thebaic tincture. And especially he recommended a volatile aromatic julep, to "retard the fatal effect."

Clearly, Rush and Currie were at opposite poles. Clearly, they would remain there. Currie would go sturdily on with his traditional, careful, cautious Cullenian procedure, developing his pamphlet into a longer work the next year: *A Treatise on the Synochus Icteroides, or Yellow Fever.* To Currie, Rush's theory and practice were alike madness. To Rush, Currie's caution was murderous.

The doctors had chosen sides.

IV

To enter a sickroom, to smell the foul, close odors of dissolution, to expose oneself constantly to infection, was a formidable task. The doctors were in grave danger, and well they knew it. Dr. Shippen left town after the meeting of the Fellows on August 25. His friend Kuhn, as soon as he recovered, fled to Bethlehem. The illness of M'Ilvaine, Carson, and Wistar alarmed all their colleagues. Dr. John Morris in Pearl Street was infected. So was Warner Washington, Rush's student. Dr. Young on visiting his first patient became dizzy and faint.

Dr. Physick came down with fever, and was treated by William Potts Dewees, who accepted Rush's regimen. Dewees bled Physick twenty-two times, taking 176 ounces of blood, a procedure both men regarded as responsible for Physick's recovery. No such chance was given Rush in the case of Dr. John Morris. He entered that young man's room just as he expired, and "his excellent mother rushed from his bed into my arms, fell upon my neck, and in this position gave vent to the most pathetic and eloquent exclamations of grief that I have ever heard. I was dumb, and finding myself sinking into sympathy, tore myself from her arms, and ran to other scenes of distress."

Happily, Rush noted that his friend—his invaluable friend—Wistar was mending. But two other doctors were stricken the day John Morris died, and the whole city, as well as the physicians, grew sad as they thought of the tragic case of Dr. Hutchinson.

The enormous Port Physician, "one of the best of men" in Charles Biddle's language and by general consent, had taken the infection late in August, just after handing his letter to the Health Officer. He was treated first by Kuhn, until Kuhn himself fell ill. Then Dr. Currie took charge, and called Benjamin Smith Barton and another young man to assist. They followed Currie's mild system. Rush was convinced this treatment was fatal. Hutchinson, he recorded, "continued to object to taking my medicine and was supported in his obstinacy by two young Doctors who had obtruded themselves upon him."

Though Hutchinson apparently recuperated, on the remission of the fever he sank very low, and died on the evening of September 6.

So well was he on Tuesday last, that he considered himself out of danger [a fellow physician wrote] and on the following morning, drew up a state of his case, for publication. His relapse was owing to his coming down stairs, and the fatigue of his going up, by which his nose got to bleed, and discharged beyond his strength.

"Hutchinson—the good, the benevolent, the patriotic Hutchinson, is no more!" exclaimed Republican Andrew Brown in

the *Federal Gazette*. Federalist Ebenezer Hazard wryly remarked that his death "demolished the Democratic Society."
Only forty-one years old, amiable and generous, known for his
charities and his republican opinions, warm advocate of the
French cause, Hutchinson had preserved a moderate and sensible attitude throughout the fever, albeit at times a confused one.
Benjamin Rush deplored the moderation as much as the confusion. Indeed, Rush did not share the general affection and respect the city entertained for the Port Physician. He described
Hutchinson as "vauntful and malignant" and reported that the
gigantic doctor, on first learning of the mercurial purge, had
threatened to give Rush a flogging. Of course, Rush was misinformed. Such vanity did not belong to Hutchinson's character.
But Rush felt the rejection of the new medicine, even at the cost
of his life, had been just one more act of jealousy and animus on
Hutchinson's part.

It was remarkable, he added, with some exaggeration, that
Hutchinson had "denied the existence of a contagious fever in
our city for above a week after it appeared among us, and even
treated the report of it with contempt and ridicule. The reason
I fear was, the first acct. of it came *from me*. . . . Poor fellow!
He died as well as lived my enemy."

Rush opened his Bible to the Fifty-second Psalm and read of
the mighty man boasting in mischief. "God shall likewise destroy thee for ever, he shall take thee away, and pluck thee out
of thy dwelling place, and root thee out of the land of the living."
This was, he thought, the very truth with the melancholy loss
of Dr. Hutchinson.

To all the doctors, Hutchinson's death was a sober, disturbing warning. Even a Fellow of the College was not immune
from this pestilence. The doctors told each other alarming stories of the manner of his infection. One said that Hutchinson
had put a young women into a coffin with his own hands, after
she died at his house. The abstemious Rush averred that the
physician's seizure came from his dining too heavily with Jefferson down at Gray's Ferry in the open air. But a much more

vivid report was circulated generally about the city. Hutchinson had assiduously attended the poorest victims in the most squalid districts. After his death people told how, with his attending student, he called on an ancient pauper woman in a wretched tenement, how when he opened the door of the sickroom a stench so foul poured forth that his student ran clear out into the street, but Dr. Hutchinson went in, opened the windows, and sat some time with the dying woman. That night he had the fever.

The good Doctor had not been dead a day when Governor Mifflin (just as he left for the Falls of Schuylkill) appointed James Mease and Samuel Duffield his successors, jointly, as physicians of the port. At once they began the inspection duties Hutchinson had not been able to perform. Mease told Rush his fortune was now made for life—he succeeded to Hutchinson's practice, and to his public office. Other young doctors were similarly supported in their labors by the knowledge that money was rolling in. Anyone who could pretend to the name of physician was in great demand.

But no one had much time for finances. By Friday, September 6, when Hutchinson died, all the doctors except Rush were nearly defeated, and Rush was now in a position from which he could not retreat. The older men remembered the fever of 1762, making the inevitable comparisons with their present disaster. Rush had been a student then, Redman his teacher. Redman, frail, retired, famous, was still available. To him the doctors turned.

With all their doubts in mind, with all their fears and disputations, with Hutchinson's death and Rush's startling theory, with Currie's steady formulary, and above all with the conviction of desperate urgency, the Fellows of the College of Physicians assembled on Saturday, September 7, in an extraordinary meeting. Before them came their venerable president. John Redman at seventy-one was the dean of Philadelphia medicine. Under him many of the physicians present had taken their first training. Short, stocky, animated, a kindly man respected and loved, Redman was a figure to inspire confidence and rededica-

tion. He had prepared a paper on the nature and cure of the
yellow fever of 1762—prepared it by studying the notes in his
daybook of thirty years before, by looking over records Rush
had kept as a student, by talking with "an ancient woman and
others" whom he remembered having treated then. The Fellows
listened hopefully.

Redman described the previous epidemic, its scope and
spread, its symptoms which distinguished it from the cholera
morbus and to some extent from the present plague. He described its effect on the system:

a stagnation and corruption of the bile and the contents of all the
abdominal glands, dissolving the blood and other fluids, and thereby
depraving and debilitating all the functions of life . . .

Redman remembered that the doctors had avoided bloodletting and emetics as too violent, rejected laudanum as too
upsetting, the bark as too depressing. The treatment most successful had consisted of moderate salts and numerous cordials,
antiemetic powders, simple mint, cinnamon, snakeroot, camphor
and theriaca, rhubarb, a plaster to the stomach, herb tea, lemonade, and fresh punches. These kept up the perspiration, kept the
bowels open but not loose, and, so the Doctor said, had resulted
favorably. He had used many other remedies in particular cases,
but no mercurials or antimonials—this from ignorance, Redman
confessed, and expressed the hope that the subsequent enlarge-
ment of the medical science would not deter their employment
now. Customarily, vinegar had been used extensively, to avoid
contagion. Doctors had rubbed their faces with it before approaching the patient, and Redman had also kept tobacco in his
mouth while in the sickroom.

Dr. Kearsley's use of saline purgatives, Redman said, had
come from his having encountered a practical observation in
"an old author." It was, he urged, "a hint to us not to neglect
the practical observations of even antiquated authors. . . . Yea,
tho' we may with some reason, from the enlightenment of medical science since, smile at their mode of theorizing . . . let us

rather pay all due respect to their memory and give them all the credit we can. . . ."

The College must have listened to Redman with mixed feelings. He had no nostrum or cure-all. He had only the healer's injunction to work devotedly, gently, and with faith. What was inexpressibly discouraging, even frightening in his relation, was the dreadful thought that so much was still to come. The plague of 1762 had begun in August and lasted into December; it had taken as many as twenty lives a day. Now it was only the seventh of September, yet already the mortality was greater than it had been in 1762, and there were at least twelve more dismal weeks ahead. Nothing but frost or heavy rains could kill the disease.

There was only one hope. Dr. Rush, Redman observed, had recently made known that a combination of mercury and jalap used at the beginning of the fever in large doses would evacuate the stomach and intestines at once, and would prepare the way for curative remedies. This strong medicine some had opposed, but Redman was willing to support his former student. He had always favored bold practice. Use the great purge, he enjoined, but use neutral salts along with it. And, he seemed to say, rely on nothing.

Panic

*The distresses of these times cannot be compre-
hended, except by those who was present and could
know the real situation of the inhabitants. Fear
seemed to absorb all the finer feelings of the heart.*
— CHARLES WILLSON PEALE

ALL the medicines in the pharmacopoeia—the doctors seemed
determined to use them all—had not power enough to arrest
disaster or erase the horrid scenes presented in these first two
weeks of September. Terror and a numb dismay overwhelmed
people. The poorest in spirit abandoned themselves to primitive efforts at self-preservation, sometimes forsaking the simplest decencies of human relationships. In the continual failure
of the doctors even the bravest men lost hope. The city sur-
rendered to a coarsening fear.

The very aspect of the disease was frightening to look upon.
Patients had a brilliant, ferocious look, their faces dark with
blood, their eyes sad, watery, and inflamed. They sighed constantly, their skin was dry and obscenely yellow. After September 10, Dr. Rush noted, a new characteristic became universal: "the determination of blood to the brain." Laymen
learned to recognize the disease on sight, and the sight was
ghastly.

Horrors were common, but none the less horrid. They were
consuming of the spirit, profane, atrocious, repulsive. The tales
people told were of a fantastic spectre: a husband married
twenty years deserted his wife in her last agonies. Wives fled

from husbands, parents from children, children from parents. Masters hurried servants off to Bush Hill on the slightest suspicion of the disease, servants abandoned masters; "less concern was felt for the loss of a parent, a husband, a wife or an only child," Carey wrote, "than, on other occasions, would have been caused by the death of a servant, or even a favorite lap-dog."

Rich merchants who had given daily employment to dozens were abandoned by wives, children, friends, clerks, and servants, with only a Negro left in attendance, if that. The poor with no attendants and no money for medicines suffered dreadfully. Seven out of eight who died were of the poor, and of these a third at least died simply from want of proper treatment, Carey estimated. Many of them perished "without a human being to hand them a drink of water, to administer medicines, or to perform any charitable office for them." Bodies were found lying in the streets. A man and wife were discovered dead in bed, their little child between them still sucking at its mother's breasts. A woman, seized in labor just as her husband expired, crawled to a window and cried out for help. Two men went in from the street but arrived just in time to see her die. Midwives —those who remained in the city and escaped the plague—were unable to meet all their calls, and charged exorbitant rates.

A servant girl started off to her home in the country but was taken sick on the road and returned to town, where no one would take her in. A Guardian hauled her to the Almshouse in a cart, only to have her refused admission. The Guardian offered five dollars for a night's lodging for her, but no place was found; she died in the cart. Children were wandering in the streets, their parents dead at home. A laborer with the improbable name of Sebastian Ale hired out as a gravedigger. An old man, he had long since lost the sense of smell. He opened a grave to bury a wife with her husband who had died a few days before. His shovel struck and broke the husband's coffin, from which emitted such an "intolerable and deadly stench" that Sebastian Ale sickened immediately and in a day or two died.

A woman whose husband had died refused a coffin for him as

too cheap. She bought instead an elaborate and expensive one, only to die herself the next week and be buried in the cheap box she had rejected. A Water Street man discovered his wife *in extremis,* and fled the house to avoid infection. Next morning he came back with a coffin he had purchased for her, only to find her recovered, while he himself died in a few days and his wife found a use for the coffin. One night a sailor lay drunk in a Northern Liberties street. Examining him from a discreet distance, some neighbors concluded he was dead, and called the carter. When he felt himself dragged by the heels toward a coffin the sailor awoke from his stupor and startled the carter by prodigious howls.

These were the stories people told. The sights they saw were pitiably worse. As mosquitoes buzzed in the damp heat, the citizens looked about them on a wretchedness they could not cure, the cause of which they did not know. The very air of the city was now infected, Rush wrote. Contagion would carry at least clear across the street.

Whole families were afflicted. Stevens the saddler was the sixth of his family to die; four persons in the household of George Hammond, the British Minister, were ill. William Young had ten in his house down at one time. The Reverend James Sproat, his wife, son, and daughter all died, as did Michael Hay, his wife, and three children, David Flickwir and five of his family, Samuel Weatherby, his wife, and four grown children. From one house more than twenty persons were carried away, some to Bush Hill, some to the grave. In other families five, six, eight, ten, and in Godfrey Gebler's family eleven, died.

All other diseases were forgotten. Indeed, Rush and some of his colleagues assumed no others existed. The fever was "a monarchical disorder," Rush told his wife on September 7. It had quite chased influenza from the city. He treated every illness as if it were the fever.

Yet in spite of the desperate panic some general observations were made. Oliver Wolcott noticed that every time the wind blew from the northern quarter patients improved and fewer new cases occurred. But whenever the wind shifted to the south, blowing across the rivers or up from the swamps and meadows below the city, the number of sick multiplied, and the fever was more fatal. Therefore, he concluded, the malady increased with heat and diminished with cold.

Other thoughtful persons noticed that French exiles seemed to be immune. The doctors explained this to Mathew Carey in various ways. Some said it was because the French despised danger, others that the French made frequent use of *lavements* at all times, which purified the bowels, discharged foul matter, and removed costiveness, "one of the most certain supports of this and other disorders." The French themselves sometimes said it was because they did not, like Americans, eat unripe fruit. Neither Carey nor Rush counted the cases among the French and Santo Domingans treated by the foreign doctors.

To young people the fever seemed particularly fatal—everyone noted that—and to housemaids, to tipplers and drunkards and corpulent persons, to prostitutes, and to the poor who lived amid filth in airless tenements. Among the old and infirm, on the other hand, the disease claimed fewer victims and, on the whole, women were less susceptible than men. In wide, airy streets not many died, but in crowded, dark, and stagnant alleys no house remained uninfected. And frequently there were the "walking cases"—those who protested they were well, who would not lie abed, who went about their business as usual, grim spectres with yellow skin and bloodshot eyes, until suddenly they fell dead.

With the breakdown of civil government, distribution of food to the poor ceased almost entirely, so by the middle of September people were starving. Scenes so frightful, and the general despondency, caused all sorts of exaggerations. One Philadelphian wrote a friend in Norfolk that half the inhabitants had fled and the remaining were dying in such abundance "they drag them away, like dead beasts, and put ten, or fifteen, or more, in a hole together. All the stores are shut up."

Exaggeration at such a time was deplorable. For those who looked closely there were many comforting signs. The impetus of trading still carried people to business every day. Such stores as remained open did very well indeed, and those who had farms or country places to rent or carriages for hire, the two notaries who "protested for the banks," the makers of coffins, the apothecaries, bleeders, and doctors attained a sudden prosperity. Even ordinary business processes went on to some degree. A new countinghouse opened in Dock Street—almost unbelievably, the proprietor was named Blight. James Calbraith & Co. advertised for sale a shipment of elegant British goods just arrived. Samuel Benge, fresh from London, set up opposite the State House as an upholsterer and venetian-blind maker. M. Blanchard continued his amazing aerial experiments from the back yard of Governor Mifflin's closed house. And in the less infected residential district Folwell's Young Ladies' Drawing School commenced its fall term.

Ships continued to arrive—one day thirty came in, thirteen of them from the West Indies. The papers, doing what they could to calm the people, stopped publishing so many obituaries. "Amen" in Brown's *Federal Gazette* wrote praising the citizenry for their clean-up campaign, particularly the clerks of the markets who had removed "putrid sheep's heads and other noxious offals." He observed that areas formerly offensive were now "delightful to the olfactory nerves."

II

Yet such reassuring signs did not go very far, particularly as the number of deaths mounted higher and higher. Doctors turned away patients by the dozens. And no nurses were to be had. With the first recognition of the disease, it became impossible to hire anyone to attend the sick. Soon people noticed that Negroes seemed immune (a conclusion they would have to revise later) and this report gained such currency that a number of colored people, completely untrained, were persuaded to take service in infected houses. Rates offered for nurses and attendants, black or white, were exorbitant, and the Negroes were blamed for it. Nurses demanded three or four dollars a day. They exacted it "with the utmost rigor from starving families," Mathew Carey said, and then they failed to do their duties. The publisher charged further that Negroes even plundered houses. Ebenezer Hazard observed that since nurses received board and room in addition to their fees, their pay was as high as congressmen's. Vicious stories were circulated about the Negroes. Many blamed them for carrying contagion, or preying upon the diseased.

Later, when Negroes proved as susceptible to the fever as whites, some of their leaders intimated that the report of their immunity had been only a wily stratagem of white people to persuade them to serve. This was not true. Actually, Negroes were not infected (or at least, not seen to be) until the disease had raged a full month. The Negroes had no better friend in all America than Benjamin Rush, and Rush certainly thought them immune until after the middle of September. He wrote his "dear friends" Richard Allen and William Gray of the African Society, pleading that since God had granted them special exemption from the disease, they had a particular obligation to come forward and attend the sick of all ranks. The newspapers carried similar appeals, and in the first week of September the Negroes responded.

Now Philadelphia's Negro community, of over twenty-five hundred people, had never been dearly cherished by the city. There were great champions of the people of color, of course— the Reverend James Sproat, Dr. Rush, the leading Quakers; and the Abolition Society was the model for all such societies in America. But the Negroes, even the more than two thousand freedmen, had few economic opportunities, and no social equality. Graduation from the African School did not mean that a Negro could rise in business or the professions or in the world of affairs. It only meant he could bear his limited destiny more philosophically. Negroes were day laborers, domestic servants, or tradesmen in a small way. Women were cooks and laundresses. There were outstanding personalities among them, but the vast majority of the black people lived insecurely on the verge of starvation.

Yet from among these, the poorest, most despised of the city, came some of the most heroic figures of the plague year.

The elders of the African Society met on September 5 and decided they must see what the Negro inhabitants could do to help the stricken white citizens. Two by two, they set out on a tour of the city. Absalom Jones and Richard Allen went to a house on Emsley's Alley where they found a mother dead, a father dying, two small children hungry and frightened. They sent for the Guardians of the Poor, and moved on. That day they visited more than twenty families. Other Negroes did likewise, and afterwards all the elders came together again to tell what they had seen.

Next day Jones and Allen called on Mayor Clarkson to ask how the Negroes could be of most use. The Mayor received them gratefully. These two Negroes were the first volunteers that had come to him, the first Philadelphians prepared to accept the plague and overcome it. Most of Clarkson's Federalist friends had fled, and nearly his entire civil service, but the city was at last producing new and courageous leaders from its humblest people. The Mayor sent an announcement to the papers: anyone wishing help should apply to Jones and Allen of the African Society.

Absalom Jones and Richard Allen were men dismayed by neither the terrors of the pestilence nor the injustice of public slanders. Their lot as Negroes in white America had formed them to endure both. Born in slavery, they had earned their freedom—earned it by the long, hard way of purchase. Absalom Jones had learned to read in slavery. He bought a spelling book. He worked in his owner's store, packing and delivering goods. Somehow he learned to write. Somehow he attended night school. He borrowed money, bought his wife's freedom, saved a few more dollars, bought a home. Then, at the age of thirty-eight, he purchased his own freedom. He continued to work in the store, he prospered. He even built two houses and rented them. He was now a man of forty-five, large, rotund, impressive.

Richard Allen, thirty-three, had made his way in the world sheerly by the strength and appealing beauty of his spiritual force. Born a slave to Chief Justice Chew, sold as a child to the Stokeleys of lower Delaware, he experienced a conversion at seventeen, became a Methodist, began preaching. His mother, brother, and sister followed him to the new church. He learned to read and write. Finally for a great sum he purchased freedom. He drove a salt wagon, labored in the fields, preached Methodism to all who would listen—to white and black alike—in Delaware, Pennsylvania, Maryland, and Jersey, in cities, in towns, in forest glades of the frontier. At twenty-six he came to Philadelphia. He preached at St. George's Methodist Church, he worked as a cobbler.

The illiterate and poor among the Negroes needed help from their own. Absalom Jones and Richard Allen founded the Free African Society in 1787—first organization of Negroes, for Negroes, in all America. It was a social organization, a non-sectarian society designed to give mutual aid to members in sickness and to care for widows and fatherless children. Its leaders were Negroes of education and substance who worshiped with Jones and Allen at St. George's Church.

Then one day an appalling thing happened at St. George's. In the midst of prayer, white trustees of the church advanced on the kneeling Negroes and ordered them to go sit in the gallery. One tried to pull Ab Jones to his feet, saying he could not kneel there. Jones said, "Wait until the prayer is over, and I will trouble you no more." But the trustee beckoned to another white to come and help him. The prayer ended, the Negroes talked together. They had helped build this church. Allen's preaching had been immensely popular, with the whites, too. This insult, this manhandling, they could not bear. They decided to leave. Led by Jones and Allen, the colored worshipers went out from St. George's, and, said Allen, white people "were no more plagued with us in the church."

Absalom Jones took one group with him, to establish St. Thomas', first Episcopal church for Negroes in America. Jones became deacon, then Bishop White ordained him priest, first Negro rector in the country. Richard Allen established a Methodist church, the mother church of all Negro Methodism. Eventually he rose to be first Bishop of the African Methodist Church of North America.

All Philadelphia knew Jones and Allen in 1793. All Philadelphia knew their piety, their honesty, their ability. Now all Philadelphia was to learn their courage. The African Society, intended for the relief of destitute Negroes, suddenly assumed the most onerous, the most disgusting burdens of demoralized whites.

The Society supplied nurses on demand, and when carriers of the dead were needed, Jones hired five Negroes to gather the bodies, put them in coffins, and haul them to the graveyards. Jones and Allen themselves shared this grim business, on regular schedules. They secured others to transport the sick to Bush Hill. There, they found things so deplorably inadequate and disorganized that they reported back to the elders of the Society. The elders asked the Mayor if he would not liberate certain Negro prisoners from the Walnut Street Jail on condition that they would serve as nurses at the lazaretto. The Mayor, confident of Jones and Allen, freed the prisoners, and those Negroes labored at Bush Hill with conspicuous devotion. Dr. Rush spoke with warm pride of his friends "Billy Grey and Ab Jones." He began a course of training for them. He directed them where to procure medicines, showed them how to bleed and when, asked them to send for him or his pupil Edward Fisher if they needed help. Jones, Gray, Allen and their helpers bled above eight hundred persons following Rush's prescriptions.

What time they could spare from carrying the dead, Jones and Allen devoted to visiting the sick, purging, and bleeding. For Dr. Rush they made careful notes on all their cases, and on the

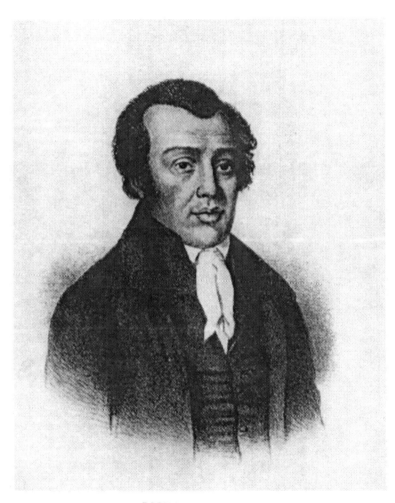

RICHARD ALLEN

appearance of bodies immediately after death. The whole city watched them every day as they made their rounds, every night as they drove the dead carts. And, of course, the city shunned them as infected, vilified them as predatory. No conduct, however heroic, could expiate the original sin of a dark skin. Doctors who opposed Rush's great purge and copious bleedings attacked the Negroes for practicing his cure, and even citizens who bid highest for their services accused the Negroes of profiteering, plundering, extorting.

Actually the African Society was going in debt for its pains. Of course, there were some Negroes who plundered and extorted. Two thousand people of any color are not all saints. But the venal ones were not those supplied by the Society. The elders ultimately found the hire of carriers and purchase of coffins had been much more expensive than the small income received for interring the dead and burning the bedding of patients. The African Society ended the year with a deficit of £177/9/8. Jones and Allen rebelled at the aspersions of Mathew Carey. He, they observed, had first fled the city, then returned to profit from his tracts on the fever.

Mayor Clarkson was apprehensive, however, and called the two Negro leaders in to discuss the high prices. Jones and Allen told him they buried the poor with no charges at all; they never fixed rates, or asked for pay. They left this entirely to the stricken families. Yet sick people all over the city offered fantastic sums for their services. A few cases of payment were gaining public notice far beyond their importance. Clarkson realized that little could be done. He did, however, arrange that public authority should pay the charges of carrying the dead, and published notices in the papers asking people to add nothing to this in the way of remuneration. It had no effect, of course; but at least it offered official support to Jones and Allen in their attempt to keep prices down.

By mid-September, Negroes were beginning to take the disease. Overnight, it seemed, great numbers were seized. "If the disorder should continue to spread among them," Rush wrote, "then will the measure of our suffering be full." He cared for many, noting some curious differences between white and black patients—Negroes were more infected when it turned cool, no Negro ever hemorrhaged as whites did. Soon Richard Allen himself fell very ill, and called Dr. Rush. Jones for a while was left with the whole burden of the dead.

Absalom Jones and Richard Allen were not men to let insults and abuse go unnoticed. The accustions Carey and others had made were slurs on the colored race too base to stand unanswered. When they found time, Jones and Allen wrote a book about the plague and their experiences in it. They wrote with deep feeling and with honesty, these former slaves, founders of churches, social reformers. Their slender little volume was one of the most affecting records produced that whole tragic year. *A Narrative of the Proceedings of the Black People, during the Late Awful Calamity in Philadelphia, in the Year 1793: and a Refutation of Some Censures, Thrown upon Them in Some Late Publications* was printed by William Woodward at the sign of Franklin's Head. It reported in simple, unornamented prose the gruesome scenes the Negro carriers had witnessed.

They had seen many white people acting "in a manner that would make humanity shudder." They saw a white woman demand and get £6 for putting a corpse into a coffin. They saw four white men extort $40 for bringing it downstairs. They discovered a white nurse pilfering buckles and other valuables of Mr. and Mrs. Taylor, who died together in one night. They found the white nurse of an elderly lady who had died (a Mrs. Malony) lying drunk, with one of the patient's rings on her finger, another in her pocket. And they passed a white householder who threatened to shoot them if they carried a body by his house. Soon he himself was dead and in their coffin.

Sometimes Negro carriers were called to bury a patient whom they found still alive. Sometimes they found no one in the house of a dead person but helpless children. They picked up boys and girls wandering aimlessly on the streets and took them to the orphanage. Once a Negro saw a white man push a woman out of a house. She staggered to the gutter and fell there insensible. The black men found she was far gone in fever, and took her to Bush Hill.

Colored people exhibited, their leaders wrote, "more humanity, more sensibility" than the whites. A poor Negro named Sampson went from house to house caring for the sick and taking no reward. When he himself fell a victim of the fever, none of those he had helped would aid his family. Sarah Bass, a colored widow, went from one sickroom to another, taking only what was offered her. Mary Scott nursed for half a dollar a day, refusing more when she could have it—in gratitude, a white patient settled on her a pension of £6 a year. One elderly colored woman, when asked what her price was, answered "a dinner, master, on a cold winter's day." A young Negress refused to take money because God would see it and afflict her with the disorder, but if she nursed for nothing he would spare her. Caesar Cranchal, Negro, nursed without pay, declaring he would not sell his life for money, even though he should die— which he did.

Such examples of Negro heroism Jones and Allen proudly set down. They were "sensibly aggrieved" at the charges against them. Many of their people had given their time, their energies, their substance, their very lives in service. They did not deserve the calumny heaped upon them. And the two great leaders were manfully aware of the purity of their own conduct. Mayor Clarkson could bear witness to their labors, and Dr. Rush, and thousands whom they had aided, perhaps saved, and thousands whose dead they had buried.

And, indeed, many others. In Boston, a newspaper published a poetic "Eulogium" to Absalom Jones and Richard Allen:

> Brethren of Man, and friends of fairer clay!
> Your Godlike zeal in Death's triumphant day
> Benignant Angels saw—they lent a smile,
> 'Twas temper'd with the dew of sympathy divine. . . .

III

Not all white people were unmanned, of course. True, some men noted for their bravery behaved less than gallantly. Commodore Barry retired to the country and would permit no one from the city to come near his house. Captain Sharp, who had fought with distinction in the Revolution, one night heard his wife complain of feeling ill and, thinking she had the fever, jumped out of bed and shut himself in another room where he died in a day or two, though his wife recovered. It did not pass unnoticed that the intrepid Commodore Thomas Truxtun left the city. And Charles Biddle observed his clerk, a Hessian veteran of the war, weaken in his determination to stay at work when he saw twelve "corpuses" passing his house at one time on the way to Potter's Field.

Others, however, rose to nobility. "Amidst the general abandonment of the sick that prevailed," Carey wrote, "there were to be found many illustrious instances of men and women, some in the middle, others in the lower spheres of life, who, in the exercises of the duties of humanity, exposed themselves to dangers, which terrified men, who have hundreds of times faced death without fear, in the field of battle." When the disaster was over, many of these were dead. Ministers were as busy as the doctors, visiting the sick, comforting the bereaved, and feeding the hungry. The young Guardians Wilson, Sansom, and Tomkins labored endlessly day and night, and the stewards of the Almshouse attended to business without a break, doling out their supplies for the poor throughout the city.

Heroism of the few only pointed up the fearfulness of the many. Fear, said "A. B.," weakened the nerves, debilitated the constitution, depressed the mind. Fear could actually cause the fever. So could great exertion. Biddle believed that Captain Sharp had been "frightened into fever," and Rush found that the men who manned the fire engines, sprinkling the streets to lay the dust, were often overcome.

Fear could certainly cause disasters of more tangible kinds.

A demoralized city is a city out of control, a city in which crime, decay, and fire are inevitable. On the night of September 7 fire broke out in Second Street below Market. It started in Kennedy's soap house, spread to Thomas Dobson's printing house and the stables and warehouses near-by. The engines came; some spirited citizens bathed their heads in vinegar, took tobacco in their mouths, and turned out to fight the blaze. It proved "one of the most obstinate fires to extinguish" that editor Andrew Brown could remember. One man in the bucket line looked at his companions on either side, reflecting that they might have come "from the gloomy chambers of debilitated friends or relatives."

Two persons were killed and several others badly hurt before the French frigate *La Precieuse* and the East Indiaman *La Ville de l'Orient* maneuvered their equipment into play and put out the fire. Republican seamen of France received for a day what praises the distrait city could spare from its preoccupation with a more general disaster, but Dr. Rush made the lugubrious note that strenuous exertions at the fire and the numerous colds taken caused many more persons to be seized with the fever. Dobson's stock of Currie's pamphlet, printed only the day before and but half sold, was burnt up; so was part of Hazard's *Historical Collections*. People thought of this as "the Great Fire in Second street." For weeks afterwards a long ladder belonging to one of the companies lay in Chestnut Street. No one was interested enough to remove it.

Panic was as contagious as sickness, as revolting as the black vomit, as formidable as death itself. There were those who remembered that a Methodist boy six months ago had predicted this fever, and years before Friend Jane Watson had told the Pine Street Meeting one First Day of the determination of the Most High against the inhabitants: He who sitteth upon the Pale Horse, He whose name is Death, would be sent through the streets of Philadelphia.

Now were visions made reality. A Marylander beheld two angels conversing with the watch at midnight, and heard the voice of Doom in Philadelphia's streets. Doom cried out in the words of Ezekiel against the modern Tyre that dwelt at the entry of the sea, perfected in its beauty by its builders. In the day of its ruin all its riches and its wares, its mariners, pilots and calkers, its dealers, and its men of war would fall into the waters. Its suburbs would shake. "The merchants among the people hiss at thee. Thou art become a terror, and thou shalt nevermore have any being."

IV

On that Saturday, September 7, members of Holy Congregation Mikveh Israel assembled in their little upper room on Cherry street. It was Rosh Hashanah, the New Year 5554, a day of mighty holiness, of awe and terror. Outside, many Philadelphians were laid in hasty graves that day, while inside Parnas Benjamin Nones, Rabbi Jacob Cohen, and all the fifty families of Philadelphia's Jewry felt the imminence of death.

They had seen the fever in their own homes. They had nursed, the sick, had endured the starvation, the lassitude, the obsceneness, and indignity of plague. Never in the fifty years of the synagogue's existence, not even that desperate time sixteen years before when Howe's army had come marching into the city during the month of Elul, had the Penitential Days brought such present griefs and fears. Sadness imbued the ancient pious words of old Amnon of Metz with a new and piteous understanding: *On the first day of the year it is written, and on the Day of Atonement the decree is sealed, how many shall pass away and how many shall be born, who shall live and who shall die, who at the measure of man's day and who before it, who shall perish by fire and who by water, who by sword and who by wild beasts, who by hunger and who by thirst, who by earthquake and who by plague . . .*

By fire, by earthquake, by plague . . . The great fire in Second Street on Rosh Hashanah tried the stricken city almost beyond endurance, and before the Day of Atonement came fantastic rumors of earthquakes: Reading, Lancaster, and Bethlehem felt severe shocks. Fugitives wrote back to the city describing them. The electric fluids of the earth, undispelled by lightnings, were restless. "Tremendous times!" Mrs. Henry Drinker wrote. "Wars, Pestilence, Earthquakes . . ."

Rabbi Cohen stayed in the city through Yom Kippur. Then he fled. It was his duty, he was told. Most of his congregation were sick or had left the city. He headed for the high and healthy country, taking lodging at Easton where he met Judge Bradford, there on judicial circuit. Bradford told him he was quite right to leave. The only protection was flight. This was an enemy to be conquered by distance, not by power. Bradford wished Rush had not started telling people to stay in the city. Of course, Dr. Kuhn's flight was a different matter, the Judge opined. It was desertion of duty, an act of cowardice.

Everyone felt the same about Kuhn's "craven flight," particularly as the need grew daily worse. Young Dr. Barton was down now, and Senator Anthony Morris was "on the verge of life." And John Barclay had to be carried home from the bank in a litter. Foreign ministers fled: George Hammond of Britain settled in Lansdowne, Don Joseph de Viar, Spanish Commissioner, took his family to Trenton, Citizen François Xavier Dupont, French Consul, fled to Bensalem in Bucks County, but not soon enough—he died there of the fever. Reports of hideous mismanagement of Bush Hill were whispered about the city. "Poor Philadelphia!" exclaimed Susan Dillwyn: "lately so full, so gay, and busy. Now a mournful solitude." Was there any prospect, she wondered, except the entire desolation of the town?

" 'Tis really an alarming and serious time," Mrs. Henry Drinker confided to her diary. She was summering in Germantown, for the Drinker house on Front Street below Race was always unhealthy in the autumn. "Our House is left, filled with valuables, nobody to take care of it—ye Grapevines hanging in clusters, and some of ye fruit Trees loaded." Reports of the plague had come out to Germantown slowly at first, but soon the city road was crowded with fugitives. They applied at every house for lodging, everywhere they were turned down. They

described the scenes in the city. Some citizens were dying of
fear, Mrs. Drinker heard. Some died on the streets, or along the
Germantown Pike. In the Drinker's neighborhood in the city
lived a slatternly old hag named Clarey. She sold oysters in a
cellar in Front Street below Elfreth's Alley. Clarey lost her
senses and wandered out of town. Someone found her dead on
the road. Hosts of rumors flew about—that five Negroes were
arrested for poisoning pumps, that hundreds of French soldiers
were marching on Philadelphia from New York, that all manner of disasters were impending.

Elizabeth Drinker went regularly to Meeting in Germantown,
where every First Day she gathered more news, of a nursing
mother refused admission to the hospital dying in a cart, of a
fugitive from the city lying either drunk or feverish in a field
near the eighth milestone (no one daring to go near him to find
out which), of the deaths of dozens of friends and acquaintances,
of a trench dug in Potter's Field for the pauper dead. Loaded
wagons jamming the Germantown Pike in continuous line from
the city made a melancholy sight. Dr. Lusby, who came out
with his family from Second Street, told the Drinkers the frightful numbers of the dead.

By Tuesday, September 10, the deplorable state of the city
was reflected in every line published on the fever. There seemed
not space enough in the newspapers to relate all that was happening. Advertisements called for creditors of decedents' estates,
and hawked the familiar nostrums. An appeal to bankers urged
that all notes be renewed so the respectable inhabitants could
leave the city—a live debtor was a better risk than a dead one,
the writer seemed to think. Half a column was given to an
earnest plea for removing the sick poor to Bush Hill as soon as
they were infected; another urged masters to send servants to
the country and urged that all infected people should be segre-
gated and kept together. Since the city government had arro-
gated so much power to itself, it might do that, too. The emptiness of the streets, the furtive burials by night, the flight of
thousands were all described.

But the worst news of the tenth was a tiny three-line item: "This morning, the PRESIDENT of the United States, set out from town, for Mount Vernon."

To his close associates, there was nothing particularly surprising about President Washington's departure. It was his custom every year to go off to Virginia in the early fall and stay until near the time for Congress to meet. Fifteen days during the latter half of August the newspapers had carried the familiar

NOTICE

All persons having accounts open with the household of the President of the United States, are requested to present them for settlement before the first day of September ensuing.

But this year the fever lent a disconsolate aspect to the President's move. Washington was officially the symbol of state, personally a figure to inspire confidence. His robust dignity, his commanding presence, gave the streets an air when he rode them, and made the city proud. His departure was noticed everywhere.

General Washington had had a miserable summer. His neutrality policy was difficult and unpopular, Jefferson was resigning; his personal secretary, Tobias Lear, had left. Alexander Hamilton was his principal support in public matters, but Hamilton came down with the fever. He was stricken on September 5, Mrs. Hamilton soon after. At once the Secretary of the Treasury called Dr. Stevens, whose method proved so successful that Hamilton sent a letter to the papers about it. He hoped, he said, to quiet "that undue panic which is fast depopulating the city, and suspending business both public and private." He wished to rouse the courage of the citizens to save lives, to prevent pain. He praised Stevens, whom he had known from their common boyhood in the West Indies, and announced that the Doctor would communicate his method either individually or in the papers before he left for New York on the next day. The Secretary told all who would listen how efficacious Stevens' cure was.

In Philadelphia Hamilton's illness became a controversial issue, because the Secretary so specifically opposed Dr. Rush and his method, so wholeheartedly endorsed Stevens' cure. In the rest of the nation his case had a different importance, for in the tense political situation Hamilton was the key figure. In every American city, anti-French partisans waited anxiously for word of "Col. Hamilton and his Lady." When his recovery was announced, letters of gratitude and relief from the most distant places appeared in Brown's *Federal Gazette*. For a while the Secretary's illness was the biggest news story of the capital city.

Public interest did not secure special privileges for the Hamiltons, however. When they left town they were shunned as infectious, refused admission to New York, had to go on up to "Green Bush" opposite Albany. There they were obliged to stay until all five physicians of Albany town trooped across the Hudson, examined them, pronounced them in good health and not likely to bring the Philadelphia pestilence to their fellow citizens.

Hamilton's support would have helped General Washington deal with neutrality matters, with Citizen Genêt, with other compelling problems. But even the presence of Hamilton that first fortnight in September could not have brought the federal government to life, for as a matter of obstinate fact public administration had come almost entirely to a standstill. Clerks in the departments could not be kept at their desks, and even heads of departments were (as Washington put it) finding "matters of private concernment which required them to be absent."

Six clerks of the Treasury Department had taken the fever, three of the Post Office, seven of the Customs Service. The Post Office Department simply shut up shop, moving the local mail service to the University building. Oliver Wolcott, Comptroller of the Treasury, tried in vain to preserve the routines of his department in spite of Hamilton's illness. He moved his family and office out to Falls of Schuylkill, to "Smith's Folly," a huge house Provost Smith of the University had built some years before. There he sought to assemble his staff. He wrote to five clerks who had fled to New York, demanding they return at once and get to work. But the clerks wrote back with wondrous excuses—the air was bad, they had no information of the fever, they had no friends in town to open their houses and send out beds and mattresses, they were not sure the government would pay their extra expenses. Wolcott was helpless. He could not in conscience demand that they endanger themselves by returning.

One Treasury clerk stayed at work, however. He was Joshua Dawson, of the Register's Office. His job was import tonnage and duties on spirits. Dawson continued at his Arch Street home, even though his little daughter died. Every day a courier came in from Wolcott, received a letter from the conscientious Dawson, and rode out again to the Falls. It was unsafe, Dawson thought, but necessary.

Public papers were locked up in closed houses when the clerks left. Postmaster-General Pickering and Attorney-General Randolph were off on an Indian treaty; their departments quickly fell apart, and they found nothing but confusion when they returned. President Washington had no one to inform him or bring him reports, none to advise or confer with him. The federal government had evaporated. No point could be gained by staying. He determined to speed his departure.

"It was my wish to have continued there longer," he wrote Lear; "but as Mrs. Washington was unwilling to leave me surrounded by the malignant fever wch. prevailed, I could not think of hazarding her and the Children any longer by *my* continuance in the City the house in which we lived being, in a manner, blockaded, by the disorder and was becoming every day more and more fatal. . . ."

He instructed Secretary of War Knox to send by every Monday's post concise information of the disease and its progress. He recommended removing the clerks and even the entire War Office out of town, and asked Knox to give advice to his housekeeper in case the presidential establishment "should be involved in any delicacy."

"I sincerely wish, and pray, that you and yours, may escape untouched and, when we meet again, that it may be under circumstances more pleasing than the present," he concluded to General Knox on the evening of the ninth.

Next morning, the tenth, the President and Lady Washington drove down to Gray's Ferry, where they visited with the Secretary of State. Jefferson was likewise preparing to leave, he told them. He handed Washington all the papers relating to the Spanish negotiation of Carmichael and Short. These Washington studied as his coach crossed the floating bridge and rumbled along down the Chester Pike. From Chester that evening he sent them back to Jefferson with his comments. From Elkton the next day (September 11) he posted another letter to Jefferson, on Saturday the fourteenth he passed through Alexandria in the afternoon, picking up a packet of Philadelphia mail that had preceded him, and reached Mount Vernon that night.

In the critical state of foreign affairs, he had planned to stay away only fifteen or eighteen days. He took no official papers with him. But as reports of the fever grew worse he postponed his return again and again. He rode about his farms, he sat endless hours at his desk writing letters, he received friends. Not for six weeks did he leave the fresh, healthy air of Mount Vernon.

v

About the time Washington left, Samuel Breck, merchant, found it necessary to return to Philadelphia. Late in August he had gone up the river to Bristol, where his family had fled. But he had a ship loading for Liverpool at the Walnut Street Wharf and wanted to see to its clearance. On September 9 he wandered clear up Front Street from Old Swedes Church to Walnut, observing the dismal scenes of the plague. As he started back to Bristol he passed the lodgings of Vicomte de Noailles. The

Vicomte leaned out of his window and cried, "Fly as soon as you can, for pestilence is all around us!" Breck flew.

Charles Willson Peale, encumbered with his museum and a large family, could not leave. Peale's museum was famous over all America, an amazing collection of improving spectacles—paintings, stuffed animals and birds, fossils, botanic specimens, dioramas—displayed at the artist's residence at Third and Lombard. The engaging painter was, James Hardie wrote in his *Directory*, "remarkable for his ingenuity and perseverance rather than for pecuniary achievements." It was an observation all the artist's friends could agree with, for his twenty-five-cent show was far from profitable. It was absorbing to Peale, however, and to his children—those extraordinary children with their astonishing names—Raphael, Angelica Kaufmann, Rembrandt, Titian, Rubens, and baby Sophonisba Angusciola.

With his wife and some of the children, Peale had spent several weeks at Cape Henlopen collecting birds for the museum. They first learned of the city's disaster when the vessel bringing them up the river was warped into the dock in early September. The painter had trained one of the Santo Domingan refugees as a frame maker, so he had been directly in contact with the reputed carriers of the disease. He shut himself and his whole entourage in his house. The birds they had collected for specimens they cooked and ate—it saved going to the market—and the artist spent his time happily classifying his collection of American minerals. He sprinkled his family and all the furniture liberally with vinegar. Several times a day he marched somberly from room to room firing off a musket charge to fill the house with acrid smoke.

Little Rubens Peale, sickly all his nine years, had been supplied with a large amount of foul-tasting medicine by Dr. Hutchinson, the family physician. When that good man died, Rubens was delighted. He destroyed all his medicines, and from then on was his own doctor. To his father, Hutchinson's death was a cruel blow, however, for soon Mrs. Peale contracted the

fever. She had experienced a disagreeable smell in the garden.
Dr. Mease came twice, took a little blood the second time. But
then he also fell ill, and Peale undertook to care for Betsy himself.
For two weeks he did not remove his clothes. He administered
barley water, laudanum, spread vinegar all around, purged and
bled according to the prescription Dr. Rush published in the
newspapers. Betsy recovered, and Peale himself survived a mild
attack, but he dwelt in constant fear.

Fear, indeed, was in everyone's heart. "An universal trepidation benumbed people's faculties," Carey wrote, "and flight and
trepidation seemed to engross the whole attention of a large
proportion of the citizens."

Yet fear itself had to have an end. As the days wore slowly
on, people became accustomed to the desperate scenes about
them, accustomed even to the obscene and disgusting facts of
disease. The heroism of a few induced an element of courage
in many. The need for workmen brought out volunteers, first
Jones and Allen, then others; and though there was no national,
state, or city government left, the Mayor served as the symbol
of calm, orderly procedures. Panic burned itself out. It was
replaced in most hearts by a calloused, blunted acceptance of the
horror, and by the determination to live with it.

A community cannot maintain panic long. Its people, in the
ordinary course of surviving, develop such mechanisms of resistance as will first meet, then conquer, the operation of fear.
In the first half of September, Philadelphians had been wasted
by panic, but in the latter half of the month they were to pull
themselves together. September 15 was the watershed of the
plague. After that day, the pestilence would no longer be a terror
without pity. It would be a fact to be confronted, and overcome.
Even though the disease grew steadily worse, even though
deaths mounted to ever higher numbers, the citizens were about
to find resources within themselves to develop a program of
control and achievement.

Panic had reduced the community to its basic components.
Among these components was the quality of leadership. The

fever was, as everyone knew, not yet half over. But from September 15 on, panic would meet its match in the leadership of three men—in Dr. Rush's serene confidence, in Stephen Girard's organizing genius, in Matthew Clarkson's cool and resolute determination.

These were the leaders who would refuse to fear fear. These were the men whose examples would bring the city out of its fantastic defeat.

"*This Excellent Physician*"

SEPTEMBER 15–30

*The different opinions of treatment excite great
inquietude— But Rush bears down all before him.*
—HENRY KNOX, Secretary of War, September 15

THE weather remained cool and dry, even pleasant, though
there was not enough rain to lay the dust, and the drought persisted. Only once in September did the temperature go above
86 degrees, twice it dropped in the night to the forties, yet the
fever was not abated by the cool weather. Indeed, the death rate
in the middle of the month suddenly doubled, and from its new
plateau began another steady increase. On September 16, sixty-
seven were buried; on the seventeenth, eighty-one; for the next
three days over sixty, then on grim Tuesday, September 24,
ninety-six. The average for the last fifteen days of the month
was nearly seventy a day.

These figures represented only burials, not numbers of cases.
Of the total sick there were no estimates. No one could, or
dared, guess how many of those who had not fled were ill. Yet
in the face of these daily tolls Dr. Benjamin Rush became ever
more enthusiastic over his great purge and copious bloodletting,
ever more confident of the correctness of his new principle of
medicine. Some doctors were horrified at his practice, but Rush
continued to bleed and purge, continued to believe himself in-
creasingly successful. So surely did he write and speak, so con-
temptuously treat nature, so casually did he dismiss personal
misfortunes, so effectively scoff at his colleagues, that people
began to flock to his waiting room and beg for his treatment.

114

Assailed with many patients where formerly he had been assailed with many doubts, Rush was expansive and jubilant. Now he entered that state of self-delusion which was to shape, first with praise, then with blame, his permanent reputation in the history of medicine.

At the beginning, every doctor who adopted his cure Rush welcomed, and expected that success would win all others over. Even when one of his own students, young Warner Washington, fell ill, Rush's confidence did not abate. "The new medicine bears down all opposition," he declared on the sixth. Deaths, he averred, studying his list of patients, were chiefly of poor people who had no doctor, or of respectable people in the hands of quacks or enemies of mercury. He stopped entirely advising people to flee the city, now enjoining them to stay home and send for "a mercurial physician." "My medicine," he told Julia, "has got the name of an *inoculating powder,* for it as certainly and as universally deprives the yellow fever of its mortality, as inoculation does the small pox."

Yet Benjamin Rush, even with all his confidence, all his belligerency, all his myopic disregard of obvious facts, could not help realizing that the disease everywhere increased. On September 8 he was called to more new cases than he had time to count. His chair was arrested in both Arch and Third streets; he was dragged to six bedsides; people stopped him in the streets to say they prayed for him. And on the eighth he won a victory—Dr. Parke, the "most bitter enemy and calumniator" of mercury, adopted the great purge publicly.

"Thro infinite goodness I am preserved not only in health," Rush wrote Julia, "but in uncommon tranquility of mind, never elevated, and never but twice depressed, and each time by a sudden paroxysm of sympathy with the distressed. The fear of death from the disease has been taken from me, and I possess perfect composure in the rooms of my patients."

Yet more and more died; and after Parke no other doctors joined Rush's lists. Indeed, other doctors began to publish cures of their own in the papers, and to attack mercury. At first, Rush

received their strictures calmly enough. "Some of my brethren
rail at my new remedy, but they have seen little of the disease,
and some of them not a single patient," he wrote on the fifth.
"Most of the publications in the papers come from those gentlemen. They abound in absurdities and falsehoods." He was learning more about his medicine as the days passed. It would not
cure, unless it produced *"large, black* or *dark* coloured evacuations," and it must be taken early. He also noted that cooler
weather brought a change in the character of the disease. But his
convictions did not falter. He formed the habit of saying, when
called to a new patient, "You have nothing but a yellow fever!"

Nothing but a yellow fever! Rush believed by September 10
that if only all the physicians would follow him, no further
deaths would occur. Mease, Penington, Griffitts, the two Glent-
worths, Parke, were all mercurial men now, but Dr. Kuhn was
still opposing the great purge from his retreat, and Hodge followed him, and Currie, and Linn, and many others. Hence,
Rush believed, the persisting mortality; hence the tragedy, the
disasters. He was ready to lay it all at Kuhn's door.

If only, he prayed, his colleagues could see the truth—the
simple truth of mercury and jalap. "Besides combatting with the
yellow fever, I have been obliged to contend with the prejudices,
fears and falsehoods of several of my brethren," he complained,
"all of which retard the progress of truth and daily cost our city
many lives." How could people still believe Adam Kuhn, after
he had taken refuge in Bethlehem?

Especially after they saw what the loyal doctors endured?
"Hereafter my name should be Shadrach, Mesach or Abed-
nego," Rush wrote Julia on the tenth, "for I am sure the preservation of those men from death by fire was not a greater miracle
than my preservation from infection of the prevailing disorder."

All around him, even in his own home, the pestilence struck.
Everyone, sick or well, had yellow in his eye and dilated pupils,
everyone had a fast pulse. All the rooms in his house were
infected. He was full of contagion himself. "My breath and
perspiration smell so strongly of it that a lady with more truth

than delicacy complained to me of it a few days ago," he confessed to Julia.

Living with the Doctor at Third and Walnut were his ancient mother; his sister; Marcus, his colored servant; and Peter, a mulatto boy of eleven. Five pupils were serving him: Warner Washington and Edward Fisher of Virginia, John Alston of South Carolina, John Redman Coxe and John Stall of Philadelphia. Washington was a relative of the President, Coxe a grandson of old Dr. Redman. Warner Washington concealed his infection from Dr. Rush. He took a room in the country; on September 11 he died, "a victim to his humanity," Rush wrote.

The other pupils moved in at Third and Walnut, to aid the Doctor at all hours. Between the eighth and fifteenth of September, Rush saw and prescribed for a hundred to a hundred and twenty patients a day. His pupils each saw twenty to thirty more. They had to refuse fifty or sixty calls a day. Even while they ate, patients were admitted, interviewed, the mercury and bleedings prescribed. "We lead a camp or wilderness life," Rush wrote. They gave up meats and wine, existed wholly on broth, milk, and vegetables, drank nothing but water. Fisher and Coxe were both yellow and feverish, but they treated their complaints "with as much indifference as a common cold."

The house was saturated with infection. Soon Rush and his pupils gave up even elementary precautions. They threw away their vinegar rags, and when there were not enough bowls for his pupils to use, the young men would take patients out to the front yard on Walnut Street and bleed them as they stood in the open air. The blood flowed freely on the ground, dried and putrified there, stank hideously, drew flies and mosquitoes. "From this source," Rush observed, "streams of miasmata were constantly poured into my house, and conveyed into my body by the air, during every hour of the day or night."

By September 12 Rush began to tire. He was sleeping only three or four hours a night. His sleep was restless, interrupted by profuse sweats. "These sweats were so offensive, as to oblige me to draw the bed-clothes close to my neck, to defend myself from their smell." He gave up broth, whereupon the offensive faetor of the sweats disappeared; but still he could not sleep.

"When it was evening I wished for morning; and when it was morning, the prospect of the labours of the day, at which I often shuddered, caused me to wish for the return of evening."

Then the inevitable happened. Late at night on September 14 he found a patient in need of bleeding. Rather than send for a barber at that hour, Rush performed the operation himself. It overheated him. He shivered as he rode home in the cool night air, and was feverish until morning. Next day he arose, met his first patients, then at eight o'clock lost ten ounces of blood. Immediately afterwards he went in his chair to visit between forty and fifty cases. At one house he had to lie down a short while, at another he was overcome at the sight of a dying friend.

Back home that afternoon he was taken with a violent chill and seizure at two o'clock. He called Johnny Stall and young Coxe to him, placing himself entirely in their care. If he sank below consciousness, they alone were to prescribe for him. He took the mercury purge and went to bed. In the evening he took a second powder, and lost ten more ounces of blood. He drank weak tea and currant-jelly water.

Next day, the sixteenth, he bathed in cold water for some time. At eight o'clock he admitted persons seeking advice to his room, and received his pupils' reports. Unfortunately his four young men could not visit all his patients and theirs too. Several cases died for want of their attention. But Dr. Rush, with mercury and bleedings, was so much improved that he slept better that night than he had for a whole week previously.

"Thus you see that I have proved upon my own body," he wrote Julia, "that the yellow fever when treated in the new way, is no more than a common cold."

All through the city the news of his illness spread, and brought a new apprehension. Rush's death would mean more than his loss. It would mean the end of his system, the failure of his cure. Letters poured in, from all quarters. Even Samuel

Powel, lying sick across the Schuylkill, wrote twice and sent fresh grapes. But Dr. Rush was far from dead.

On the seventeenth he was the first person up in the house, and was well enough to come downstairs. He sat in his parlor, prescribing for over a hundred people, he sent his young men out among his patients to bleed and purge. "Like old General Harkemar I am fighting the disease thro' them, upon my stumps," he wrote.

On the nineteenth he hired a carriage and resumed his visiting, though he was still weak. His fever hung on, and a cough. He had trouble climbing stairs, his hands were hot. The stench of sickrooms made him dizzy. From now on, Dr. Rush was not fully well, whatever he said, or whatever the newspapers published to the contrary.

Yet he continued to treat as many as a hundred and fifty cases a day, and in the evening to write to doctors, to pour his heart out in wonderful letters to Julia, to record his observations in notebooks. He continued to bleed and purge, to wonder that other doctors would not follow him. And he continued to recoil from the horror of death.

Around the city, his friends were dropping daily. Rush saw "the great and expanded mind of Dr. Penington shattered by delirium" just before he died. The young Quaker had been "dear and beloved" to Rush, "like a younger brother." And in his own home tragedy struck frightfully.

Just as he himself was recovering, Johnny Stall fell ill. Rush put him to bed at once, in the back bedroom. Soon Edward Fisher collapsed, and was laid in the front room. The house was a hospital, Rush wrote. John Alston gave way next, in his room at Mrs. Wilson's, whose daughter he had been caring for both as suitor and as doctor. Even John Coxe was drooping. Then Marcus, the colored servant whom Rush had trained to mix powders, spread blisters, and give enemas "equal to any apothecary in town," yielded to the disease. He was bedded down in the doctor's laboratory.

It was fantastic. By September 22 Rush had lost one apprentice (Washington), had two more and a servant ill in his own home, and John Alston very low near-by. Coxe was up and around—he did his duty, Rush observed, "with a spirit that he never showed before." And the mulatto boy Peter helped. He was "to us now, a little host." The Doctor even sent Peter to see patients.

But all would die for want of care. Rush appealed to Jones and Allen, who procured two colored nurses. They moved in, to nurse Stall and Fisher.

Suddenly Rush discovered that Johnny Stall had deceived them all. That brilliant youngster—poet, painter, musician, scientist—had administered Rush's cure to hundreds, but in his own case he rejected it. First Fisher, then Coxe had given him mercury purges, but Stall had not swallowed them. He lied about his evacuations, said the purges had worked. Rush and Coxe tried to force the mercury down his throat, but he spat it out. He was delirious, Rush concluded. In spite of five bleedings, he sank below hope. At noon on September 23 he died.

Rush loved him deeply. Forever afterwards the Doctor kept by him the fragment of a letter Johnny Stall had begun to his father, unfinished when the pen fell from his hand. "You must excuse me," Johnny had written, "as I am doing good to my fellow-creatures. At this time, every moment I spend in idleness might probably cost a life . . . so many doctors are sick, the poor creatures are glad to get a doctor's servant. . . ."

"Scarce had I recovered from the shock of the death of this amiable youth," Rush wrote, "when I was called to weep for a third pupil." On the twenty-fourth John Alston—"my dear boy Alston"—expired. Alston, a gentle, handsome lad from Carolina, had caught the disease, apparently, from his beloved Miss Wilson. Dr. Rush could not be found until many hours had passed, yet Alston refused to allow anyone else to bleed him. "Life and death often turn upon the application of a remedy at an hour or a moment in this ferocious disease," Rush said sadly. Alston had seemed to be recovering. Then one day just after taking mercury he drank a whole pint of cold water. At once, he began to puke, retched terribly, and died in fearful convulsions. The black nurse should have been more careful, Rush thought. "Such accidents must often happen when the sick are nursed by blacks ignorant of their business, and frequently asleep or out of the room."

Edward Fisher, fortunately, was recovering. Five copious bleedings and the purge again and again had saved him. And Marcus mended. But on September 26 Rush was assaulted with repeated calamities. The day began with a call to Dr. Redman. The fine old man was gravely ill, in the greatest danger. At 12 o'clock his grandson, John Redman Coxe, Rush's only remaining apprentice, was struck down. He was taken to Dr. Redman's house from which Rush had just returned. "I followed him with a look," the Doctor wrote, "which I feared would be the last. . . ." The afternoon brought a call from Samuel Powel.

At two o'clock Rush's sister, who had complained for several days, took to her bed; and that evening his mother was likewise stricken.

Rush was now completely alone: Washington, Johnny Stall, and Alston dead, Coxe ill, Fisher still abed, his mother and sister down—September 26 was the day of his greatest trial.

That evening, finished with the business of the day, Rush sat before the fire in his front parlor, his mouth dry and black from the mercury, his hands hot, his body weak, his cough racking and painful. A "solemn stillness" pervaded the whole city. "In vain did I strive to forget my melancholy situation by answering letters and putting up medicines, to be distributed the next day among my patients." The colored Marcus, out of bed for the first time, crawled from the laboratory and came to the parlor door. Rush bade him sit by the fire. ". . . but he added," said the Doctor, "by his silence and dullness, to the gloom, which suddenly overpowered every faculty of my mind."

The weakness of humankind flowed in upon the weary Doctor as he kept the long night watch in his fetid chamber. Yet when dawn came on, a wind stirred. The sky lowered, and a few drops of rain fell upon the parched roofs and dusty streets.

Rush roused himself. Even in the extreme moment of his life, the work of another day must be done. He opened his Bible to Psalm 121. It was, said his Book, "A Song of Degrees." *I will lift up mine eyes unto the hills, from whence cometh my help. My help cometh from the Lord. . . . The Lord is thy keeper: the Lord is thy shade upon thy right hand. The sun shall not smite thee by day, nor the moon by night. The Lord shall preserve thee from all evil: he shall preserve thy soul. The Lord shall preserve thy going out and thy coming in from this time forth, and even for evermore.*

A Song of Degrees. He was, he wrote, "much comforted." Benjamin Rush began a new day. He had passed his personal crisis. He was ready again to bleed, to purge, to proclaim his great new principle in medicine—to tell more patients, "You have nothing but a yellow fever."

He was ready to give his confidence, his faith, his moral strength to all men.

Panic is cured, not by reason, but by firmness. Rush was firm in his course, firm in his assertions; and the very firmness of his presence in the shuddering city brought hope, courage, and reassurance to many who had been paralyzed with panic. That he was wrong, tragically, disastrously, frightfully wrong, everyone was not to realize for more than a century, nor shall we ever know how many lives his errors cost. But the courage he imparted to others was as healing as his purging and bleeding were probably destructive, and the spiritual sores of the city began to mend under his energetic if dubious ministrations.

II

Physicians, Andrew Brown wrote, were public property. It was the nature of their calling to face danger. People looked up to them as to a kind of Providence, with a faith it was exquisite cruelty to destroy. No physician in the knowledge of men had ever so perfectly met the requirements of this ideal as Benjamin Rush was meeting them now. Jones and Allen declared they were "willing to imitate the Doctor's benevolence, who sick or well, kept his house open day and night, to give what assistance he could in this time of trouble." Judge Bradford said of Rush, "He is become the darling of the common people & his humane fortitude & exertions will render him deservedly dear." Fugitives in Easton drank his health, prayers for him ascended from congregations all through the country.

Dr. Rush became the popular hero of the plague. And as though the simple heroism of his staying and serving were not enough, legends and fables began to circulate about Rush, to make his service all the greater. In one of the most colorful of these stories, the Doctor smilingly admitted, there was enough of the truth to make it acceptable. It was told how one day the inhabitants of Kensington saw his familiar coachee cross the bridge into their town, where there were great numbers of victims. Knowing he must return by the same route, a huge crowd rushed to the bridge and barred his way. They begged him to visit their homes, or at least to tell them how to treat the fever. There were several hundred. Rush, without stepping down, threw back the top of his curricle and addressed the multitude "with a few conciliatory remarks." Then he cried out in a loud voice, "I treat my patients successfully by bloodletting, and copious purging with calomel and jalap—and I advise you, my good friends, to use the same remedies!"

"What?" called a voice from the crowd. "Bleed and purge every one?"

"Yes!" said the Doctor. "Bleed and purge all Kensington! Drive on, Ben!"

III

Now the tragedy of the Yellow Fever of '93 is, of course, that the mercury purge and copious bloodletting were erroneous, probably fatal, treatments. So the riddle of the fever of '93 is a question of character analysis. The riddle is: how could the brilliant Benjamin Rush have come to believe as he did, and with egregious obstinacy stick to his belief?

Rush was, a contemporary wrote, "wonderfully entangled in

the web of his honest sophistry." It was sophistry of his own making. He was not following old errors; he was consciously, proudly departing from them into new and greater errors of his own. He was not misled by others; indeed, others whom he should have respected argued forcefully against him. He was not justified by his observations; his observations, even as he records them, show how wrong he was. Yet as he watched death a thousand times that fall, he continued to believe himself right, his cure successful, his patients helped. He grew ever more courageous, ever more determined, ever more convinced.

Actually, Benjamin Rush was neither saint nor sprite, and his occasional resemblance to either was purely coincidental. He was an intensely human person, unusually aware, unusually vivid, with a highly developed sense of the dramatic. His physical energy was considerable, his restless mental energy prodigious; he was a ready victim of every trap self-deception could lay, a personality who found his security in the good opinion of others, a man invincible save by his own enthusiasms.

A more candid nature would have recognized at least by mid-September that the amazing theories of bleeding and purging had only the slenderest basis in literature or in practice. Mitchell's old folio had come to his hands when Rush was in deepest despair, almost without hope. In such desperation even reasonable men will seize at any frail support. But to discard every canon of scientific caution, and in one week to proclaim desperate remedies a new principle in medicine; further, to insist upon the principle against all opinion without verifying experience, and to continue such insistence until it became a fixed idea—became indeed the exclusive doctrine of a whole career—this was to pass beyond the sphere of reason. How could Dr. Rush have moved so rapidly, so wholeheartedly, into his looking-glass world?

The Doctor was no mere theorist. He was a keen recorder and analyst of what he saw. Yet first of all he *was* a theorist, and as September moved on, his abundant resources for adjusting facts to his theories were wearing thin. Rush might have abandoned his theory, accepted the burden of error, and started over again. But he was a human being, not a demigod, and being human he took the part of the theoretical philosopher—he ignored the facts and kept his theory. He recognized no error, except in others.

It is a still more difficult matter to explain how anyone he treated survived Rush's ministrations, particularly when we learn that he, like his contemporaries, thought there was about twice as much blood in the human body as there really is. Rush was willing to take as much as a quart of blood at a time, and to repeat this process several times in two or three days. When his great purge caused the bowels to bleed, he thought this merely an additional benefit supplementing his venesection. The more blood lost, the better. He urged that bleeding be continued at intervals until "four-fifths of the blood contained in the body are drawn away." Dr. Physick was bled twenty-two times, Dr. James Mease lost 162 ounces, Dr. Griffitts (small, frail, weakened by previous illness) bore seven bleedings in five days. Now Rush believed that the total volume of blood in the average person amounted to twenty-five pounds or a little more. Actually, it is less than half of that. Imagination staggers at the thought of Rush, his pupils, his colleagues, his favored Negro nurses, and all those lay people who followed his printed directions in the papers, prepared to draw four-fifths, or twenty pounds, of blood from patients who contained no more than twelve.

Rush was the most complicated of men, a personality who almost defies explanation. The evidence of his senses should have shown him the error of his treatment. Yet he persisted in believing his method a cure. Why?

One reason was his own recovery. He had proved the method "upon his own body." Yet by his own careful evidence, he was bled only twenty ounces in twenty-four hours, took only two of the powders—a far milder regimen than he prescribed for others.

More fundamental reasons supported his confidence. One was his religious faith. Another was the praise of distant doctors. A third was his daily experience with the citizens of Philadelphia in that fall of '93. In these elements lay the answer to the riddle of Benjamin Rush—in them also lay the moral problem of the great plague.

IV

Dr. Benjamin Rush approached religion with the same contentiousness he took to medicine and politics, indeed, to his whole life. His religious allegiance had been erratic: first Episcopalian, then Presbyterian, then Universalist, then once again Episcopalian; now lately, because St. Peter's was going high church, he was returning to Presbyterianism. Too independent to remain long in one sect, too conventional to break from all, Rush had wandered from church to church, periodically excited by precious points of Protestant polemic.

Through all his denominational meanderings, Rush had preserved a steady, aggressive piety. He performed morning devotions, read daily from his Bible; he sustained a lively sense of the personal immanence of God. At Princeton and Edinburgh he had absorbed religious influences without absorbing religious doctrines; and in spite of his scientific association he had always resisted the dogmas of deism, that religious refuge of the scientist who purported to discover God through the study of nature. Consequently, Rush had neither the inordinate respect for nature characteristic of one part of his intellectual generation, nor the precise definition of God in doctrine characteristic of another. Yet his piety was both sincere and unaffected; moreover, it was a sort of piety particularly useful to him, for the not unusual reason that the object of his pious devotion was so entirely a creation of his own, responsive to the changing needs of his emotions, a God uninhibited by doctrine. Rush's piety was like looking into a mirror.

Thus the American Sydenham, beset on one side by the hosts of disease, on the other by his fellow physicians, found his God an ever present help this tragic autumn. One day, September 22, when three and thirty were buried in Potter's Field before midafternoon, he was reminded that the words of the funeral service were reversed for him: in the midst of death he was in life. "But O! by how tender a thread do I now hold it. I feel as if I were in a storm at sea in an open boat without helm or compass. My only hope and refuge thou knowest O God is in thee!"

Divine Providence, he wrote, daily delivered him from infection—surely it was a miraculous intervention. And Providence singled out him, and him only, among all Philadelphia doctors, to accomplish the heavenly purpose. "I am thankful for this great privilege," he told Julia. "It is meat and drink to me to do my Master's will. He loved human life, and among other errands into our world, he came 'not to destroy men's lives but to save them'!"

Jesus, he reflected, had performed his labors with a body much weaker than his: "I profess to believe in, and to imitate a Saviour who did not *risk,* but who *gave* his life, not for his friends, but his enemies."

Because, he declared, of the prayers of his wife and friends, "purified and accepted thro' the mediation of a gracious Redeemer," he was twice recovered from the fever himself, and through faith was enabled to bear the horrible conditions of his life. He prayed continually, and begged others—his family and acquaintances, his patients, at one time the whole village of Princeton—to pray for Philadelphia. "Indeed, I have thought that all good Christians should *sit, walk, eat* and even *sleep* with one hand constantly lifted up in a praying attitude to the Father of mercies to avert his judgments from us. O! that for his elect's sake he would cause the time of our sufferings to be shortened!"

Only such pious faith, renewed by such continual pious exercises, could have sustained Rush in his courage and confidence. Only such faith, with its inner conviction of righteousness, its element of direct inspiration, its unquestioning assumption of special providence and superiority, could have blinded him to the facts about him. However great its cost to others, Rush's sturdy piety convinced him of the truth of his discoveries. God would not have revealed false doctrine. Nor would God have tried him lightly, burdening him with the fever and with intransigent opponents, without great and serious cause. His was a proper Christian situation, for God's will was done on earth, "as much by pestilential contagion, and ignorant physicians as it is by the songs and praises of saints and angels in heaven."

Confidence bred of such faith was able to bear scorn and obloquy, and to ignore defeat. Rush was a proud and sensitive man. He frequently winced under the castigations of his colleagues and detractors. But even those attacks which wounded him most he could answer (when recovered from his hurt) by reflecting on his divine mission. It never occurred to him that he might be wrong.

It occurred to others, however. His Princeton classmate Ebenezer Hazard fell ill, and sent for Rush. The Doctor bled him twice, plentifully, and administered mercurial purges. Then Hazard firmly refused further bleedings and mercury, and sent for Dr. Hodge. Rush was incensed; he wrote Julia when Hazard recovered that the patient had *survived* the remedies of Dr. Hodge, but *his* early purging and bleeding had laid the foundation of the cure.

Hazard's account was somewhat different, and would have pained Rush had he read it. The historian wrote his friend Belknap that Rush was boasting lustily of his successes, while at the same time three of his own apprentices had died. When he first called the Doctor, Hazard continued, Rush took twelve or fifteen ounces of blood, and gave a powder; next day eight or ten ounces more, and another powder, third day more bleeding and purging. Hazard then felt his own pulse, and objected to further bleeding as unnecessary. This opinion, said the Doctor, was one of the most dangerous symptoms in the case: "the disorder was extremely insidious; the case extremely critical; not a moment to be lost; send for the bleeder directly. In the mean time, take this pill; and, if that does not operate in one hour, take this. You must be glystered to-day; but, if you are not *bled* to-day, I shall not be surprised to hear that you are *dead* tomorrow." Hazard declared he would lose no more blood; Rush declared he would no longer treat the case, and stamped off, leaving the patient to die. Hazard "took some bark, to strengthen his stomach; drank a little wine, extraordinary, to enrich his remaining blood; and ate nourishing food in *small* quantities, but *frequently.*" He recovered.

This experience with Rush's method was shocking to the reflective Hazard. He regarded the famous Doctor, his old friend, as anything but a divine messenger.

"He is a perfect Sangrado," he observed, "and would order blood enough to be drawn to fill Mambrino's helmet, with as little ceremony as a mosquito would fill himself upon your leg."

v

Pious faith in his own rectitude would not have been enough, by itself, to support Rush in his confidence, had all his experiences belied him. But actually—and nothing is more curious about the whole plague year—Dr. Rush's personal experiences everywhere confirmed him. Not the deaths of his patients, of course, but all the other personal experiences of his days. Responding to his courage, inspired by his abundant vitality, his kindness and optimism, elevated by his evocative faith, people adored Dr. Rush. They stopped him in the streets to tell him so, they wrote letters of gratitude and joy to him and about him, they composed poems in his praise. They sent to him in dismal fear, and he comforted them. Many called him their savior. They bore the same testimony elsewhere, publicly. Such people could not be wrong.

Of course, some wrote the Doctor in criticism. One man described his cure by a mild saline purge, and others wrote giving advice of their own. Matthew McConnell on the west bank of the Schuylkill occupied the hours while his wife was in labor composing a letter that urged the Doctor to bathe every morning in warm vinegar. But far more numerous were letters seeking guidance and sending thanks.

No sooner, it seemed, had Rush received his inspiration and

laid down Mitchell's manuscript than doctors, former students, and friends in other cities began to seek his advice. William Gardiner of Darby, who had sat under Rush at the hospital, wrote asking what the disease was and how to treat it. Dr. Francis Bowes Sayre of Crosswicks in Jersey described the case of a woman he had lost who showed numerous petechiæ on various part of her skin, and asked Rush's opinion. A few days later her husband was seized, and Sayre wrote again, pleading for guidance as he had "exhausted the catalogue of tonics, stimulants and antiseptics."

Dr. John R. B. Rodgers from New York told Rush of the fears of that city, and the talk of quarantines. He agreed that the coffee could have caused the original fever, but asked whether additional agents of contagion were not necessary to account for the wide spread of the pestilence. Fear, he believed, was a cause of fever, and he guessed that the four thieves of Marseilles had been preserved as much because they were hardened, fearless villains as by the operation of their vinegar. He talked of whitewashing, and of removing woollen carpets.

Rush answered Rodgers, as at first he did all the others, and the New Yorker read the letter to his medical society, the members of which he declared much interested in Rush's cure—though Rodgers must have misunderstood his friend in part, for he regarded the disease as imported, and asked for news of Secretary Hamilton's recovery by the French method.

From Burlington in Jersey a friend begged information and expressed "inexpressible gratitude," and from many other quarters came similar appeals. Then, when news of Rush's great discovery began to spread, a very spate of letters poured in. Dr. Belleville, a refugee physician in Trenton, told Rush his discovery had unquestionably subdued a fever which otherwise would have "prouve very destructif." It had conquered panic in Trenton. Dr. John Griffiths of Rahway asked for the exact dosage of calomel; Rush's "affectionate pupil" Henry Colesberry of New Castle begged directions, as did Abraham Ridgely, practicing at Chestertown in Maryland, where a fugitive from

Philadelphia had died. John Bayard of New Brunswick asked Rush to write him once or twice a week, for a young man on the Philadelphia stage had died of the fever, to the consternation of the inhabitants, and before his death had told of Hutchinson's tragic fate and Rush's great success. Bayard was sure that Rush would keep him frequently informed because of the alarm of the New Brunswick citizens. From Bristol Dr. Minnick sent for "the cure" and likewise asked Rush to give him news of his friends.

All correspondents praised Rush's humanity and courage, all committed him to God's care, all begged for help. The elegant Elisha Cullen Dick, who as a student had left Rush without permission and gone to study with Dr. Shippen, was now practicing both medicine and Masonry in a conspicuous fashion at Alexandria, Virginia. (Seven years later he would bleed General Washington in his last illness.) He wrote Rush "soliciting a correspondence" on the fever, contributing for his part an account of Alexandria's current sickness. It was all too apparent to Rush that Dr. Shippen, Dick's real preceptor, was not available for his former student's assistance. From his friend the Reverend James Muir of Alexandria, Rush learned that Philadelphia vessels were barred from the town, and that a day of fasting and prayer had been proclaimed. Dr. Charles Washington of "George Town on the Potomac" appealed to Rush "from my knowledge of your liberality as a Physician, your ability to investigate the Cause of Diseases, and your great willingness at all times to propagate useful medical knowledge." Dr. George Wallace of Elkton pointed out that his village was much exposed to Philadelphia and a refuge for the fugitives. And Sylvanus Baynton of Chatham near Fredericksburg, eulogizing the heroism and success of Rush, requested news of his brothers and sisters, his aunt and her family, of Mrs. Rush, the children, and others. He promised to expose the Doctor's reply to sun and air for some hours before handling it.

For a while Rush continued to answer these and all other letters, but soon they became impossibly burdensome, particularly when added to all the local calls upon him for the same information. Accordingly, to save himself the time of writing to country practitioners, as well as to "help the people to cure themselves not only without, but in spite of physicians who know nothing of the disorder," he published his cure in the newspapers. It appeared on September 11: as soon as you feel pains in head or back, are nauseated or have chills and fever, take one of the powders (ten grains calomel, fifteen jalap) in a little sugar and water, every six hours, until they produce four or five large evacuations from the bowels. Drink plenty of water or gruel, lie abed and sweat. After the bowels are thoroughly cleansed, if the pulse be full and tense, be bled of eight or ten ounces from the arm—more, if tension continues. Light diet, fresh air, continuously open bowels, blisters on sides, neck and head, cleanliness above all, should be your regimen.

It was a simple cure, as simple, Rush said, as the stone from the sling of David. Many people treated themselves from his printed directions, and some of the country practitioners found their questions answered. Many other people, however, were offended, among them of course Hazard, who objected to this and subsequent publications by Rush with all his venom. The Doctor, Hazard averred, "said so much about his success in the newspapers that he got a great run of business. He is apt to be sanguine (excuse the word, I do not mean a pun), and many think he carried bleeding to an excess." He noted that Rush's patients did not recover their strength as soon as others. "Dr. Rush was puffed off as an oracle by some, and, in every newspaper, 'Dr. Rush's Mercurial Sweating Purge' met the eye, like the advertisements of a mountebank. . . ."

Country practitioners, however, were not deterred from writing by Rush's publications. Indeed, they wrote all the more. "To *read* their letters alone would be burdensome at *any time,* but it is much more so at present," Rush observed. His postage frequently amounted to as much as seven shillings sixpence a day, so he tried again to answer everyone helpfully in one communication. He prepared a "short" account of the origins, symptoms, and treatment of the fever, addressed to Dr. John R. B. Rodgers of New York, which filled three columns of Brown's paper on October 7. By this time all the other doctors had delivered their opinions on "the cure," and the letters that came in were part of the argument.

From laymen, too, as well as country doctors, Rush received reassurance. Postmaster-General Timothy Pickering pronounced him heroic and unselfish; Congressman Thomas Fitz-Simons praised his "uncommon philanthropy." Attorney-General Edmund Randolph, who had found a house out in Germantown, wrote that he had studied all methods of treating the malignant fever, and had concluded that Rush's was the best; would the Doctor please send him medicines and advise what he should do first should anyone in his family be attacked? Judge Jacob Rush, the Doctor's brother, was on circuit in the north when the disorder began. On September 11 he reached Reading, and wrote Benjamin describing the influenza in Easton, Sunbury, and Wyoming. He begged the Doctor to clear up the contradictory reports of Philadelphia's fever that were rife in Reading—that is, to clear them up if Rush was sure the disease could not be communicated in a letter. "I mention this," the Judge wrote, "on Acct. of your being probably much more among the infected, than a Common person, and that any Intercourse with *you* is therefore the more dangerous."

Unfortunately Judge Rush got things a little mixed. He had heard that the late Dr. Hutchinson believed the disease was *not* imported, and in view of Hutchinson's well-known relationships with Dr. Rush assumed this opinion was wrong. He sent his brother a long argument in favor of West Indian origin. Ultimately the Doctor set him straight.

Maria Bright from New Jersey told Rush he was doing God's work. Beale Bordley, Chester County Quaker, praised his liberality, regretted the attitude of orthodox physicians, and bade Rush be confident that truth would prevail over bigotry and prejudice. Every day as he or his coachman Ben queued up at the temporary post office to get letters, Rush found more of these testimonies of his correctness and success. Each mail sustained him in his views, helped him maintain his conviction against every onslaught of fact or opinion.

Each mail, and every day's experience as well. The grief of John Morris' mother at the deathbed of her son Rush could not get out of his head; neither could he forget the speechless despair of Mrs. Meare, nor the delirium of Dr. Penington, nor the dying look of good Mr. Mervin the schoolmaster, who restlessly moved his hands and cried out, "Help me! Help me!" That last desperate look of Mr. Mervin quite threw his mind off its pivot, Rush wrote.

Scenes haunted him—scenes in which people clung to him, pleaded with him, depended on him. Once a sailor stopped his carriage to offer him £20 if he would see his wife. Mr. Sims fell upon his neck and cried like a child when Rush entered his house. Another time in Moravian Alley five people tried to stop him. He whipped up his horse and escaped as far as possible from their cries. In a Quaker family the Doctor climbed the stairs through a train of children weeping and blessing him. He gave their father a strong purge and ordered a fourth bleeding, after which (washing his mouth with Lisbon wine) he told the children there was some hope of the good man's recovery. They seized upon that word "hope," "as if a kingdom had been conveyed to them."

His only support in "these awful events which hourly pass" was the assurance everyone gave him that his remedies worked. Father Fleming, the Roman priest, told him many Catholics cured themselves from his printed directions, and the Reverend Mr. Helmuth said the same of the Lutherans. The testimony was universal, Rush thought. The great purge and the bleedings were proved. He promised, if he survived, to publish a complete theoretical account of his cure, and he believed it would be as effective against the true plague as it was against yellow fever.

From the greatest homes to the humblest, Rush moved with the impartiality of medicine. "The poor are my best patients, because God is their paymaster," Dr. Boerhaave had said once, and the epigram was dear to Rush. The poor flocked to his back parlor. He saw them before breakfast and after dinner, he prescribed for them from his couch, he went to their tenements, he even took two homeless children for a while into his own house. The poor seized upon every bit of news concerning him. It became known that he grew faint from walking and took little nourishment, so all around the city Rush found a glass of milk and a crust of bread ready for him when he entered a home.

And from the poor he went to the world's great—to Cabinet ministers and legislators, to merchants and bankers, to publishers, underwriters, and lawyers, to the French Legation, the British and to Mynheer Van Berkle, the Dutch Minister, who was very low. Van Berkle's cure was a triumph, for the Dutch statesman had been deceived by Kuhn and Currie's publications into believing he had only a common fever. Rush reached him just in time, and recovered him with seven bleedings. "Hundreds have been sacrificed by this mistake," he wrote Julia. "We have but *one*, we cannot have but *one* fever in town. The contagion of the yellow fever like Aaron's rod swallows up the seeds of all other diseases. We might as well talk of two suns or two moons shining upon our globe, as of two different kinds of fever now in our city."

Alexander Hamilton had advised Van Berkle to use Stevens' cure, and had said Oliver Wolcott would decribe it for him. Wolcott, however, was already praising and employing Rush, and so did the Dutchman. Thus was Hamilton overthrown. Rush wondered whether, if he had not been so staunch a Democrat and friend of Jefferson and Madison, Colonel Hamilton would have opposed his discoveries.

The rich and well born of America were his patients—Thomas Willing and Samuel Powel, old Mr. Meredith and his friend George Clymer, and a host of others. Robert Aitken (who had printed the first English Bible in America) called him for his daughter Peggy. John Nixon of the bank and the financier Alderman Barclay, John Oldden the merchant and, it almost seemed, the whole city solicited his presence.

One day brought an amazing summons: Mrs. Hutchinson, widow of the Port Physician, was stricken, so was her child. No one would help her. Would not Dr. Rush come? Rush went. Mrs. Hutchinson, deserted by all her husband's political and medical friends, had none to rely on but the one man her husband had endlessly opposed. Rush gave the widow and child the bleedings and purgings Dr. Hutchinson had spurned. They recovered. "Her expressions of gratitude to me for attending her, indicated a strong and delicate mind," Rush remarked.

To Third and Walnut streamed a great horde of patients, irresistible in their unanimous opinion of Rush. And to the Doctor's door came likewise servants, children, or old people bearing notes from sufferers, begging him to come, or send his students, or at least prescribe. Postmaster-General Pickering was caring for a serving maid in his home. Rush sent young Coxe to see her, but Pickering's daily notes described no progress. She vomited continually and groaned terribly, though with such "strength of lungs" that Mr. Pickering was not too fearful of her decline. Then his young son Edward caught the fever, and Pickering himself rode in to consult Rush. He nursed the boy tenderly, but in despair, writing Rush of each change in his condition. He refuses to take any nourishment at all—the miserable father noted as the end neared—says his throat is stopped. Should he force something down by holding his nose?

From George Clymer—who had signed the Declaration of Independence with Rush, Clymer the staunch, devoted patriot— daily notes began to come: his mother-in-law Mrs. Meredith is ill, and so is Mr. Meredith. Now Mrs. Clymer is seized. She has taken Rush's purge, which worked. Would Rush prescribe a second? Of course Rush would. Next day: she is much worse, and Clymer has sent for the bleeders. Is this right? Clearly it is. Clymer asks for a few of the mercury powders; he will take one himself and administer the others to his wife. She loses blood constantly, has a fever and headache; will not Rush take her in his rounds? Rush has claimed Clymer himself as a patient, but Clymer denies he has the fever—his complaint is only "a slight catching of the brain upon the least action of the body or intentness of the mind, caused by Thursday's hot sun," while his nausea comes from a sweet potato he ate at dinner. Should he take a purge? And should Mrs. Clymer have a gentle febrifuge such as Rush gave Mrs. Meredith? She is worse. Much worse. Finally a note arrives: "Let me entreat you Dear Doctor to make your visit here as early as you can."

Slowly Mrs. Clymer recovered. But her father, Mr. Meredith, suddenly suffered a relapse. Rush was sick and could not go out. Mrs. Meredith grew frantic. "For Gods sake dear Mr. Clymer procure some help for Mr. Meredith or he will die," she wrote. "I sent to Dr. Rush this morning but he neither comes nor sends. I shall go distracted if somebody does not come." Rush despatched young John Coxe to bleed and purge.

Alexander Cochran, Front Street merchant, sends his little brother around for directions: he has taken three purges and been bled fourteen ounces. His head throbs, and he has an oppression in the breast, his lips and gums are swollen, he is bleeding internally, last night he spat half a pint of blood. He is very weak. What shall he do? Soon he cannot send his brother, for the lad is sick also.

Michael O'Connor's wife and daughter are ill, and he himself experiences "disagreeable sensations." Will not Rush come? Young Mr. Coxe is fine, but Rush is their savior. And James Cresson and Josiah Coates and many others send servants or relatives to the Doctor's door with messages. They are all alike, these notes handed in by fearful, timid bearers—all alike, and all desperate. But sometimes one arrests even the much beset Doctor: on October 7 comes a simple note on a green half-sheet. It is from the Mayor. Mrs. Clarkson was seized with chills this morning, and is now unwell. Will Rush call at once? Rush goes.

Some are mere panic. In September Gifford Dally says he, his wife, and daughters were standing in their doorway when a cart passed on its way back from Potter's Field, and they received the most disagreeable smell that could be thought of. Should they take medicine? A month later the Dallys are all sick of disease as well as panic, and in every house on their street people are dying.

One writes of a daughter "verry weak & low, and most amaz-ingly yellow." Another describes his wife, seized with violent pain, chills, and fevers; she vomited a greenish bile, she took the powders as Rush said in the newspapers, they were successful. Are her symptoms of the malignant kind? All beg him to come. Mrs. Anne Engels thanks him for saving her two sons. Now her husband is sick, Dr. Annan has given a powder and salts and sent for the bleeder, but will not Rush himself come also?

Congressman FitzSimons, caring for his own business and that of many fugitive friends, must also care for children en-trusted to him. One is sick in a boardinghouse. Will Rush go to see him? Someone else writes of his sick brother, who calls for molasses beer. May he drink it? Wives, fathers, mothers, chil-dren detail cases in their families, curious symptoms, curious remedies; all turn to Rush.

Small wonder that the tragic procession brings the Doctor greater conviction and assurance, strengthens his faith. Small wonder, too, that the doubters move him to anger. When Rush was ill and could not come, Mrs. Jones gave her daughter the purge, as the newspapers said. Then she called Dr. Benjamin Duffield. Dr. Duffield declared Rush's powders had "ruined" the girl—she was sixteen, and had always been regular till she took mercury.

Duffield was simply malicious, Rush believed. Malicious, and a follower of the dull Kuhn. Mercury was unpleasant, of course. It dried up the mouth, stained the teeth; sometimes it irritated the viscera. But it could not accomplish the ruin of a virgin. Duffield was like Currie, Barton, Johnson, all the rest of the confederacy, jealous, shortsighted, ignorant.

More to be trusted were the simple godly people who turned to him in loving hope—people like old Edward Penington, Dr. Penington's bereaved father, who from his own sickbed sent Rush preserved fruit and fresh peaches. Or Samuel Powel, an ever tender friend. Or valiant Samuel Coates, who called one day to offer, what no one else seemed to realize was necessary, a gift of £50. Or dear Mrs. Morris, who had other patients besides her dead son, and who begged a syringe, for she could not buy one. (Apothecaries had sent all theirs out to Bush Hill.) Mrs. Morris wrote from her house of mourning, "May every blessing which the goodness of Providence may permit his bounty to bestow be the portion of the benevolent friend of Mankind."

These were his real judges—the people. These were his real masters.

Bush Hill

SEPTEMBER 15–OCTOBER 10

I do not know when our misfortunes will end. I am off now to the hospital where so many sick are received daily that my presence is constantly demanded.—STEPHEN GIRARD, September 30

Now Dr. Rush, for all his courage (and for all his extraordinary literary style), had really no enlarged or general view of the plague. His was a particularly personal type of experience. He saw thousands of cases, both in his office and on his rounds. He formed his judgments from them, and from what his young men told him; from what Griffitts, Porter, Woodhouse, Mease, the other mercury men told him, too. But this was only a part of the plague. And seeing only a part, this "excellent physician and friend to mankind" received a distorted view of his adventures. There were those who saw all Dr. Rush saw, and more, too— who saw the problems of the Bush Hill hospital, of the orphan children, of the starving poor, of the fugitive rich, of the fleeing governments, of, in short, the whole city in decay. They viewed the plague with a larger perspective than did the Doctor. And none saw more clearly, more fully, Philadelphia's plight than the sturdy, sober Mayor.

Matthew Clarkson, like Dr. Rush, passed his personal crisis in September. The fever came very close to him. There was sickness in his own household, where Mrs. Clarkson lay gravely ill, "in a bad habit." His son-in-law Robert Ralston was the busy secretary of the Santo Domingan relief committee. And a ship from the islands brought the Mayor tragic news. His youngest child, Gerard, just twenty-one, had been graduated in medicine at the University under Rush two years before, and had gone to Basseterre on St. Kitts to visit his brother David. There, on July 30 the young doctor had died, after a short illness of the yellow fever. Early in September the news reached the Mayor.

Yet even with this burden on his mind, Clarkson continued every day at the City Hall, receiving all who came to his vinegared chambers. He watched the disruption of the life of the city. His own Mayor's Court ceased, and return day in Common Pleas found only five lawyers before Judge Biddle, instead of the fivescore who usually attended. The Coffee House closed, "all the merchants being gone to the country"; and taverns shut their doors. Meetings of every kind were postponed —the Mason's Grand Lodge Quarterly Communication, church assemblies, all sorts of corporation meetings and club occasions. The College of Physicians, in spite of their resolution to assemble every Monday, had to give up. Only Redman and Currie came on September 17, next week they were both ill. The Mayor was deprived even of organized medical support.

Mail delivery ceased. Clarkson, like everyone else, had to line up at the University every day to get letters. And printers were so scarce, business so bad, that newspapers could not continue. One after another the papers suspended—those national news-papers of the national city, The *Pennsylvania Packet,* the *Gazette of the United States,* the *General Advertiser,* the *Mail or Clay-poole's Daily Advertiser.* Of the five dailies, only Andrew Brown's *Federal Gazette* continued to appear. Somehow Brown kept going. He missed not one issue during the whole pestilence, though sometimes his paper consisted of a single sheet only. Brown's *Federal Gazette* became the city's sole means of general daily communication. Weeklies and semiweeklies closed down, including the *Neue Philadelphische Correspondenz;* Bradford's weekly *Pennsylvania Journal* died of the plague. Childs and Swaine's *National Gazette,* of which Philip Freneau was editor, alone among the semiweeklies continued, but Freneau was in a bad way financially, holding on by a shoestring. His Republican scurrilities brought no comfort to the conservative Mayor.

Clarkson listened to Dr. Rush's plea that the city provide horses and chairs for physicians and bleeders. He heard the problems of the carriers from Jones and Allen. He considered the alarming situation of Bush Hill. He worried about fire hazards in the city—closed houses were sure to burn in this drought, and at the great fire in Second Street there had not been enough buckets. He ordered all housekeepers and clerks to bring fire buckets from empty houses to the constable of the watch at the Court House.

Scenes in the streets were daily more tragic. Burials were by day now, as well as by night. Victims were never laid out. They were simply wrapped in a tarred sheet (in whatever clothes they had on), placed in coffins, and drawn to graveyards in carts or hearses—no bells, no invitations, no religious services.

And to leave the city was well-nigh impossible. Stages would accept no passengers unless they bought tickets clear to the end of the line—to Baltimore, New York, or Reading. Yet they were crowded.

Banks would not discount loans. It was impossible to borrow money. And the public disagreements among the doctors were confusing, frightening, upsetting the whole city. Dr. Thomas James, a young Quaker newly back from Edinburgh, did a strange thing which brought reassurance to no one. Having a hundred fever patients, he announced that he would take no more. The disease was mysterious, he said. It was a divine visitation. Medicine could not cure it.

But no scenes, however desperate, could make so deep an impression on the Mayor as the daily reports he received from the young Guardians, Wilson, Sansom, and Tomkins. They were all the staff he had left, and they were helpless to care for the whole city. If they were to have no assistance, they might as well give up.

By September 10 the crisis in administration had arrived. President and Governor had gone; the Mayor alone remained as the head of resistance. Philadelphia would either have to rescue itself, or the city would have to be abandoned to its dismal fate.

Faced with the impossible, Clarkson forsook the attempt to run a government without personnel. Casting all constitutional restraints aside, he appealed to the citizens directly. September 10, the same day which saw Washington's departure, saw the beginning of organized community resistance to the plague. On September 10 the Mayor published an address "To the benevolent citizens," announcing that the Guardians were "almost overcome with the fatigue they undergo." They needed immediate assistance. Would not benevolent citizens help them? Let all volunteers come to the Mayor, and he would tell them how to be useful.

On the morning of Thursday the twelfth, a meteorite fell in Third Street. Perhaps it was an omen. That day a small group of benevolent citizens, reeking of vinegar, came to the busy City Hall. They made their way through the vendors of coffins and crowd of hawkers gathered in front. They were the beginning. The Mayor addressed them; so did the young Guardian James Wilson. They told them the story of a city disintegrated. The volunteers listened, then went on a tour of the town. They came back to City Hall (all but one, that is. He did not come back, and soon he was dead). They passed a resolution: Let a general call for help go out. Let a committee be formed.

The call was published. At twelve noon on Saturday, September 14, the volunteers came together again—there were nearly thirty this time; Dr. Currie was among them. A letter from Dr. Rush was read; volunteers told what they had seen in the city; three of them had been to Bush Hill. Clarkson and the volunteers heard with dismay the report of what Bush Hill was like. The four doctors did not regularly attend, the female nurses were not qualified, there was no manager, no bleeder, eight new nurses were needed, and a large sum of money. The Guardians required a great number of people all through the city to oversee the poor, the starving, and the sick, to transport victims to Bush Hill, to give relief. A committee must be organized at once—a committee to spend money, give orders, do anything necessary, keeping accounts and reporting to future meetings of the citizens. It would be a private committee, perhaps, but it must act with speed and decision, and with authority. The citizens must govern themselves.

And so, at the meeting of volunteers on Saturday, September 14, was formed the unofficial Committee which under the Mayor's direction would gradually organize Philadelphia's resistance to the silent terror of the plague. The Committee became the actual governing body of the city. The volunteers—scarcely more than two dozen—authorized themselves "to transact the whole of the business relative to mitigating the sufferings of those that are or may be afflicted," to procure physicians, doctors, nurses, and attendants, to purchase all supplies necessary. The citizens resolved to solicit $1,500 from the Bank of North America, and authorized the Committee to appropriate money from this fund for purchases and wages.

Mayor Clarkson was chosen president of the Committee, Samuel Wetherill vice-president, Thomas Wistar treasurer, Caleb Lownes secretary. The whole Committee apart from the Mayor consisted of twenty-six men, "mostly taken from the middle walks of life." Four of them never attended. Several others were stricken, and as Clarkson wrote, "from death and other causes the business was principally conducted by twelve only."

These, with the three regular Guardians remaining, were the whole staff the Mayor now had to help him care for the city, "watch over the sick, the poor, the widow, and the orphan." They conducted their business, Carey noted, "with more harmony than is generally to be met with in public bodies." They took the place of council and aldermen; they governed as if they had been chosen to do so. From this Saturday on, the Committee meeting daily at City Hall constituted the organized administration of Philadelphia.

The Committee started its work the same hour it was formed. Three members went at once to John Nixon, president of the

Bank of North America, and put up the necessary bonds for the $1,500, which Nixon promised to have ready on Monday. Three others were named to solve the problem of carriages—carriages for physicians to get about the city, carriages for the dead. It was voted to advance money to poor families with sickness in their houses, and ten members were appointed to superintend business at Bush Hill, choose the officers of the hospital, put the place in order—all this was done in a sitting.

Saturday passed, and Sunday; various members did their tasks. On Monday the sixteenth the Committee assembled again at noon. Things began to move. A contribution of $20 was received from a citizen—favorable omen—and the condition of Bush Hill was being investigated. Two members, the merchant Stephen Girard and the cooper Peter Helm, had visited the lazaretto on Sunday and made a list of what was needed. The Committee ordered everything they asked for to be purchased and sent to the hospital. A carpenter was hired to go out and build beds (his name, curiously, was William Hamilton, the same as Bush Hill's owner), a horse was bought to serve the hospital, two men engaged to attend the cart.

These were energetic steps. They demonstrated the sincerity of the Committee. And Stephen Girard and Peter Helm, as they observed the despatch with which things were accomplished, realized that the members meant business and would support the hospital to the full extent of their means. According to their pre-arranged plan, therefore, first Girard, then Helm arose, and though they had seen the horrors of Bush Hill at first hand, they offered themselves to the Committee as managers of the pest-house.

The Committee was at first taken aback at such boldness, but immediately recovered to express admiration and gratitude. Nothing could have done more to hearten the whole city. If Washington's departure on September 10 represented the nadir of despair and panic, Girard's and Helm's extraordinary offers on the sixteenth represented the beginning of effective resistance. The Committee accepted their services. They resolved that the two men "be at once encouraged to enter upon the important duties of their appointment."

That afternoon Girard and Helm rode out to Bush Hill to begin their work, with what misgivings we can only imagine. They were symbols of the new courage Philadelphians were discovering.

II

The Augean stables which Girard, prosperous French merchant, and Helm, pious German cooper, had agreed to cleanse would easily have discouraged lesser men. Indeed, Peter Helm told his neighbor Charles Biddle that when he first made his way to Bush Hill he expected never again to return to the city alive. Both men had beheld the worst the hospital could offer, both knew the stories that had been told.

In the two weeks since August 31, Bush Hill had come to stand for all the filth, stench, and corruption of the fever. No one knew how many patients had been taken there since the four dying victims had been removed from Ricketts' circus; but the number was so great, the mortality so large, that sufferers would rather lie in the city streets than be dragged to certain death at the pesthouse. The foul odors about the hospital and in the rooms were so offensive that none "but an insensible, or an heroic mind" could bear them. Carriers arriving with a load would sometimes find their carts empty. Once a lunatic who had contracted the fever consented to be taken there, but jumped out on the way and ran off, the carter galloping after him as fast as his horse would go.

The young medical student Charles Caldwell, who served there for a while as an assistant, was obliged to eat, drink, and sleep (when he could) in the same rooms with the sick. Sometimes he lay down, exhausted and careless, on the bed with a patient, to awake in an hour or so and find his bedmate dead.

At other times, under similar circumstances, I have received from a patient, on some part of my apparel, a portion of the matter of "black vomit." And I was inhaling the breath of the sick, and immersed in the matter which exhaled from their systems, every hour of the day and night. For I was perpetually in the midst of them.

Others knew the atrocious conditions of the hospital less intimately, but with more perspective.

A profligate, abandoned set of nurses and attendants (hardly any of good character could at that time be procured), rioted on the provisions and comforts prepared for the sick, who [Carey wrote] (unless at the hours when the doctors attended) were left almost entirely destitute of every assistance. The sick, the dying, and the dead were indiscriminately mingled together. The ordure and other evacuations of the sick, were allowed to remain in the most offensive state imaginable. Not the smallest appearance of order or regularity existed. It was, in fact, a great human slaughter-house, where numerous victims were immolated at the altar of riot and intemperance.

Whose fault was it? There was no one to say. Perhaps the four doctors Clarkson had appointed—young Dr. Physick was ill part of the time, so was Leib; Cathrall and Annan could not carry the load, particularly with their enormous burden of private patients in the city. Or perhaps the Guardians, who were supposed to be in charge—but Wilson, Sansom, and Tomkins had so much to do in the city, with no help, that supervising Bush Hill was beyond them. The hospital was left to itself, to become a fantastic purgatory as more and more sick were carried to it. The scandalous conditions caused such fear that poor people would not admit they were ill lest they be taken there, yet as soon as anyone was seen to be ailing,

an alarm was spread among the neighbours and every effort was used to have the sick person hurried off to Bush-hill, to avoid spreading the disorder. The cases of poor people forced in this way to that hospital, though labouring under only common colds, and common fall fevers, were numerous and afflicting. There were not wanting instances of persons, only slightly ill, being sent to Bush-hill, by their panic-struck neighbours, and embracing the first opportunity of running back to Philadelphia.

While the scandal was bruited all through the city, nothing appeared in the newspapers about the hospital, nor did the mayor make any pronouncements. A writer in the *Federal Gazette* on

September 11 complained that no accurate information was available to anyone. How was the hospital attended, by what doctors? How were the patients received, with what success were they treated, were chances of recovery actually better there than at home? Only accurate knowledge on these heads would put a stop to the rumors and idle gossip.

Plainly, conditions were so bad that no official dared say anything. The patients, wild and determined under mistreatment, had risen against the nurses and doctors, and since no civil officer was available who would enter the place, Governor Mifflin had appointed young Dr. Physick an alderman, to enforce order and deal with emergencies. Mayor Clarkson had ridden out to Bush Hill to swear in the Doctor. He approached just close enough to be heard, and (by Physick's account) "was happy to be off as soon as possible, when the ceremony was over."

III

Stephen Girard, peering wryly out of his one eye, observed all that was going on, heard all that was said, and followed his custom of keeping silent in all his seven languages.

At forty-three, the French-born Girard was a familiar figure in the city, a merchant and importer who had lived here fourteen years. He had prospered in the Santo Domingo and French trade, but his life had been saddened by the illness of his wife, a mental invalid. This, with his partial blindness, caused him to live much to himself. Until now, Philadelphians had thought him, as one wrote, "rather a decent than an extraordinary character."

For him, neither Bush Hill nor the tales that were told, neither fetid miasmas nor mephitic effluvia, held any terrors. He was a man of business, and having been a mariner, he was neat and orderly. He detested clumsiness and inefficiency. He also detested failure. The malignant fever, "which our Escupalians treat as a plague," he insisted was neither contagious nor fatal, except as the physicians made it so. While "A. B." wrote to the papers praising those "intrepid sons of Galen who have not de-

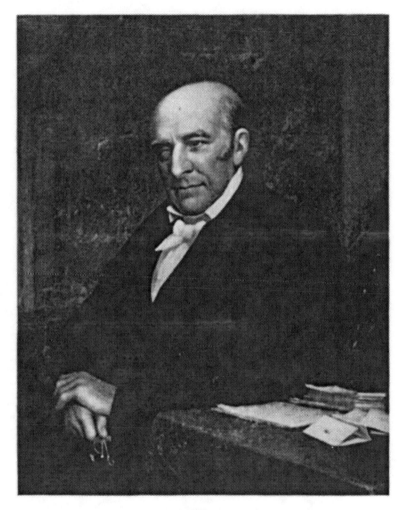

STEPHEN GIRARD

serted their posts," and begged a tear for the physicians who had died, Girard brusquely dismissed such sentimentality as nonsense, and denounced "the pernicious treatment by our doctors," which he was convinced had "sent many of our citizens to another world."

As his house was in Front Street, his business at the wharves, Girard was bound to contract the disease, which he did the last week in August. It was a slight attack and interrupted his work only briefly. Soon he was back at his desk, complaining that all the underwriters had left town, making it impossible to insure a voyage, and worrying about his brig *Polly,* last heard of at Le Cap and now long overdue. "It seems as if the misfortunes at Cap François will be fatal to me," he wrote.

Frenchmen did not die as easily as Americans, Girard dryly observed, and he speculated that if the fever raged much longer Philadelphia would have no one but Frenchmen left. Still, "the generous and benevolent Girard," as Charles Biddle called him, was neither callous nor unmoved, nor did his scorn for "the ignorance of our doctors" blind him to the real suffering in the city. When Mayor Clarkson published his address "To the benevolent citizens" praying them to help the Guardians, Girard at once came forward, as one of those "who are not afraid of death or at least who do not see any risk in the epidemic which appears to prevail." He resolved to do his whole part.

"I shall accordingly be very busy for a few days," he wrote, laconically.

In this frame of mind he turned up at City Hall on Thursday, September 12, a stocky, simple little man, calm, businesslike, determined, cool where others were excited, reserved where others were panicked. From the afternoon he and Peter Helm made their welcome offer and rode out to Bush Hill, they were in constant attendance sixty days, nursing the sick, conducting a model institution. Every day the Committee met, and every day spread upon its minutes the legend, "Stephen Girard and Peter Helm at the Hospital."

". . . for the moment," Girard wrote, "I have devoted all my time and my person, as well as my little fortune to the relief of my fellow citizens."

Peter Helm was scarcely known in the city at all. A devout, pious member of the Moravian congregation, he went about his work in homespun, wore a flat hat, used the plain speech of the pietists. He worked with his hands. His coopering shop was at his home in Race Street near Third. President Washington employed him to make things for his household—a cooler, barrels, and such things. He had none of the organizing genius of Girard, none of the executive capacity. His talents were kindness, courage, and broad human sympathy—gifts which he offered in abundance.

The new managers found actual conditions at Bush Hill far worse even than they had seemed from the outside. Needs were endless: needs of staff, of supplies, of facilities, of physicians, needs of public support. At once, managerial responsibilities were divided. Everything inside the hospital was assumed as his province by Girard, everything outside by Helm. This was a fair division of work. It gave Helm superintendence of grounds and outbuildings, carting, receiving and burying, quarters for the staff, and sanitary facilities, while Girard had charge of the rooms, the care of the sick, and general administrative duties. In his share of the work Girard was thrown into closer contact with the patients during their illness, and his tender devotion became legendary. Helm was no less effective, no less tender, but Girard's was the dominant force at the lazaretto. He at once showed himself an extraordinary as well as a decent character. Administration was congenial to him. He was, as he later styled himself, "the one who organized that institution." He encouraged the sick and comforted them, administered medicines, sat with them in their deliriums and their miseries; he performed for them the most intimate offices "which nothing could render tolerable, but the exalted motives that impelled him to this worthy conduct," he wrapped them in winding sheets when they died.

To the sufferers at Bush Hill, accustomed to none but hardened attendants or now and then a hasty visit from a doctor, the spectacle of two of their fellow citizens hazarding their lives to serve them seemed no less than a reprieve from death.

Organization was necessary immediately. Girard and Helm had a thorough cleaning done, and then allotted the fourteen rooms and three halls of the mansion to specific purposes. One room was set aside for a matron and her assistants; two were used for supplies, eleven rooms and two entry halls for the patients. Every room, apartment, and entry had its nurses. Men and women were separated, each treated by nurses of their own sex. The dying were placed in one room, the "very low" in another. A doorkeeper stood at the entrance. Every patient was provided with blankets, pillow, and sheet, with clean linen garments when necessary, and with porringer, plate, and spoon. As many as 140 sufferers were crowded into these accommodations.

On the evening of their first day the new managers reported that except for a few nurses the hospital was fully staffed with officers and attendants, that supplies were ample, "and that the business is now so far matured as to afford every assistance necessary at such a Hospital." But this report was designed for public reassurance and was scarcely accurate. Two weeks of filth and decay could not be brushed aside in one night. The managers acknowledged that they were "engaged in promoting the order of the house" and had many things to put to rights.

Helm worked out a simple though surprising system of receiving patients, which brought the hospital, a visitor found on September 20, "to a great degree of perfection." The system was this: carriers in the city would put a patient into a box, and convey him to Bush Hill. There Helm would take him out of the box and place him in a hole in the ground. He would be left in the ground until Girard and his staff had made a bed for him, with fresh linen and "every necessary cleanliness." Then he would be taken inside.

"This hole in the earth must be extremely Serviceable in imbibing the putrid effluvium, strengthening the diseased person, & doing all the offices of a cold bath," the visitor wrote.

But the hole in the earth solved only one problem. There were many other things wanted. There was no place for convalescents, no morgue for the dead before burial, no shed to store coffins, no living quarters for the staff. There was not even any water, because the pumps were out of order. The doctors were irregular in their attendance, the bestial nurses had to be turned out. The very day the managers were making their hopeful first report, the steward announced that eight patients had died, and asked the Committee for twelve coffins.

From this first day on, the Committee sitting at City Hall gave Girard and Helm every support they could. As notes came in from the managers, supplies were ordered and workmen hired. The Committee was assiduous in its part of the Bush Hill job. Because it might "subject the sick to great inconvenience to lay on the floors until bedsteads can be made," the secretary (Caleb Lownes) was ordered to go out and buy as many beds as he could find. A carter was hired for $3 per day, and a notice was inserted in the papers proclaiming

Generous wages will be given to persons capable and willing to perform the services of Nurses at the Hospital at Bush-Hill; as the end desired by establishing a Hospital at Bush-Hill much depends on good nursing and attendance, The citizens of Philadelphia will render essential service to the sick, by aiding and procuring suitable persons for this employment. . . .

More serious even than nursing was the need for regular medical care. The young doctors, Physick, Cathrall, Annan, and Leib in their busy days gave Bush Hill patients only a small share of their time. It was a two-mile ride out to the hospital, and there were many stops to make en route. Physick went out five times, Leib three, Cathrall and Annan only twice in the two weeks after August 31. They charged the city seventy shillings for each visit. Yet each was praised throughout the city for his devotion to the poor. From their fellow doctors they won another type of praise, for the autopsies and dissections they did taught physicians something of the disease they were dealing with. Annan found the brain of a patient who died after several days' fever turgid with blood. This Rush noted, and further avowed he changed his mind on important points following Physick's post-mortems; and when Physick and Cathrall published the findings of their joint autopsies in Brown's paper, medical science was edified.

Now in truth twelve visits in fifteen days was no proper care at all. The doctors, on their few trips, arrived at eleven in the morning and spent a short time among the sixty to two hundred patients at the hospital. Apparently they spent more time cutting up bodies. Even had all four been able to attend every day, they could not have examined carefully each patient in a brief visit, nor could they stay to oversee the treatment they prescribed or be sure the venal attendants followed orders. So far advanced in fever were many of the sick when they were brought in that they needed immediate attention, but Girard complained that those who arrived in the afternoon had to languish all night and until eleven the next morning before a physician would see them— and it was doubtful even then if a doctor would appear.

Obviously what was needed was a doctor in residence at all times. Girard had a man in mind. Edward Stevens was not the only physician in Philadelphia who had seen yellow fever in the West Indies, for among the refugees from Santo Domingo was Dr. Jean Devèze, "first class health officer of the French armies" at Cap François. A man of thirty-nine, Devèze like Girard refused to look upon the fever as contagious, and used the "French cure" of stimulants and quinine. Probably at Girard's urging, Dr. Devèze appeared before the Committee on the very afternoon the new managers took office and "offered his services as a Physician in such part of the Hospital as may be assigned to his care." The Committee referred the Doctor to the managers, meanwhile enquiring into his abilities and character, and proposing that if satisfactory he was to be appointed. Next morning (September 17) Girard reported that Devèze had visited the hospital, appeared "to be a professional character," had a good record at Le Cap, and seemed well qualified. So the Committee resolved that the French doctor "be desired to give his attendance at the Hospital."

Now this resolution was a bit of hedging, for the Committee was somewhat embarrassed. Devèze was actually asking for an independent command at Bush Hill—independent of the four American doctors who had occasionally called there for more than a fortnight and were following Rush's methods rather than the French cure. To appoint him "to a part of the Hospital . . . assigned to his care" would imply the Committee's censure of the four Americans, and of the medical theories they represented. Such censure the Committee had no desire to pass. Their resolution that Devèze "be desired to give his attendance" was a compromise solution that accepted his services but simply put him on an equal footing with all the other doctors.

For Stephen Girard, who had to grapple with the results of the old system, this trimming attitude was far from satisfactory. It was time for firm, decisive action. If the Committee proved spineless on this issue, it would waver on others, and Girard had need of its wholehearted support. Immediately on hearing of the resolution, he gathered Helm and rode into town. It was high noon, but the Committee had just then resolved to "continue their sittings constantly at the City Hall, until the situation of the Hospital, and the afflicted in the city shall render it proper to adjourn." A quorum could act; and before those present the managers offered it as their opinion "that a Physician should be appointed to attend constantly at the Hospital." This point Girard won. The Committeemen voted to employ a full-time doctor as soon as possible. But the appointment of Devèze to that position was too abrupt a move to carry at once. Instead, the Committee requested the four American physicians to meet with them the next morning at nine o'clock, to discuss medical care at Bush Hill.

The morning of September 18 Mayor Clarkson (having all the previous day been busy with other matters) took the chair himself, and the four American doctors—Annan, Leib, Cathrall, and Physick—appeared. The first action was the Committee's firm resolution, "that the managers of the Hospital, at Bush-Hill, have the entire direction at that place; and that they be empowered to employ and discharge such persons as they think proper." This was forthright enough. But immediately afterwards the floor was opened to the four physicians, who delivered their own opinions as to the mode of providing medical assistance.

The young doctors now had their innings. They made the most of them. They stated their case, and produced a program of four propositions for the Committee: that the physicians attend the hospital regularly every morning at eleven, that they receive two guineas each for every visit, that Mr. Graham be "prescribing Apothecary, to attend to those patients admitted in the absence of Physicians," and the further provision

That Doctors, Leib, Physick, Cathral and Annan, have the entire direction of the Hospital, to be arranged in such manner as they shall judge proper . . .

This program was clearly designed to keep the French doctor and his method out of Bush Hill. It was equally clear that it would not satisfy Girard's demands. Yet the Committee, after considering it, adopted the whole program. They had no wish to run counter to the entire College of Physicians, or to seem to prefer a Santo Domingan refugee to their own young men. Nor had they any wish to antagonize the four Philadelphians and thus lose their services.

Girard, on the other hand, was no man for the Committee to defy. He had them on a very slippery spot, for the nature of his offer and his service was such as to make it almost obligatory to accept all his terms.

Small wonder the Committee shuffled and paltered. Though they had first given the managers full charge, and a few minutes later conferred upon the doctors the same powers, now they wobbled into a greater confusion: they added to the doctors' program the provision

That a room at the Hospital be appropriated to the use of such patients as are desirous of being under the direction of Doctor Deveze . . .

This, for those who resisted bleeding. This also for Girard. Devèze was to procure his own medicines at the Committee's expense and, if he had to, provide a person to administer them.

Girard and Helm had not been present when the Committee took these curious and contradictory actions. But on assembling the next morning (September 19), the Committee found a sharp note, signed by both the managers, asserting that the program adopted would "not be productive of the benefit desired." The bemused Committee once again debated the whole issue. Mayor Clarkson was a Rushite; so were most of the fifteen committeemen present, so was young Dr. Physick, who stood before them. But this time Dr. Devèze was there too, his calm, determined person the outward sign of that question mark gnawing within each committeeman: yesterday nearly seventy burials, the day before eighty-one—perhaps the Philadelphia doctors for all their noise, for all their learned discussions in the newspapers, for all their disputations and controversies, were wrong. Perhaps these Frenchmen whom Girard knew, and who knew the yellow fever, were right.

Once again the committeemen blinked and hovered, once again compromised. They rescinded their previous resolution and passed a new one, this time separating the patients into two divisions, each division to have a different doctor, the nomination of each doctor to be left to the managers.

Under the powerful urgency of the situation, however, the Committee tried to get the question entirely settled. There stood Devèze, with the managers' endorsement; he was at once appointed to one division. There stood Physick, whom the Committee knew, and though he had not been nominated by the managers, the Committee (ignoring its own resolve) appointed him to the other.

Devèze accepted, and left at once for Bush Hill. But Dr.

Physick asked to have a night to think it over; he would not be placed in a false position.

Actually, Physick must have seen what an impossible situation it would be. Too many patients already crowded the decaying mansion. To find two rooms for the dying, two rooms for the very low, two rooms for every class of patient, simply because there were two doctors, would be impossible. It would also place two systems of medicine in an intolerably close competition. Doubtless the proposal by its ambivalence horrified Girard as well. He sent in a report, too well timed to be entirely guileless, observing that the American doctors had failed to visit a number of the sick that morning and that Dr. Devèze had accordingly called on them.

Yet, after thinking about it overnight, Physick agreed to take charge of half of the hospital, but he raised a number of questions and precipitated still another debate (September 20), which led the committeemen still further along their irresolute way: they now divided the hospital into *three* divisions, with *three* doctors, Leib being added to Devèze and Physick.

This was too much, even for the Philadelphia doctors. Next day instead of appearing they sent a letter, signed by Cathrall, Leib, and Physick, declining to serve. The Committee had feared this would happen. They despatched a messenger to inform the managers that there would be no doctors that day, and begged them to "proceed to the care of the sick and to endeavour to obtain the necessary medical aid which their situation may require." Girard, however, was well pleased. He now had what he wanted, and on the twenty-second turned up in person before the Committee to assure them they need have no uneasiness, for "Doctor Devèze is, with the assistance of the Apothecaries, fully capable of performing all the duties of the place, until the numbers shall considerably exceed those now in the Hospital."

It had taken Girard six days to maneuver the American doctors out, and get Devèze in. With his own man head of the staff, and his own theories at work, he was prepared for anything. The Committee discharged the apothecary James Graham, in spite of his protests; but some of the members were still uneasy, not the least reason being that they would be glad of a physician at Bush Hill who could speak good English and write reports, and in whose background they had confidence.

Their wish on this head was soon satisfied. No sooner had Devèze taken over and installed his own apothecaries than Dr. Benjamin Duffield offered the Committee to assist at the hospital. Benjamin Duffield, Fellow of the College, was an authority on midwifery. He conducted public lectures on that subject, and would soon add courses on the diseases of hospitals and jails, and the American practice of physic. Every committee-man knew him, and knew his background. He had been stung by Rush's sour treatment of him in connection with the "Medicus" letter; he was opposed to bleeding and the mercurial purge anyway. The chance to serve at the hospital, even under the French Devèze, he welcomed, for personal as well as philanthropic reasons.

Certainly the Committee was grateful for his service. He was thanked, and given a chaise to use. Two days later he reported back that he had visited Bush Hill, found everything there in proper order, was satisfied with the method of treatment used by Devèze, and recommended the continuance of the French apothecaries. From that time on, medical reports to the Committee came from Duffield: on September 27, the hospital was in good order, with ninety-five patients; generally those who died were hopeless cases admitted in the last stages of the disease; on the twenty-eighth, 106 patients, some recovering.

Devèze and Duffield made a good team. Twice a day they visited each patient and prescribed their medicines; their prescriptions were executed by three resident "physicians" or apothecaries. Devèze's life was not without incident. One day he was walking hurriedly from town (committees could resolve carriages but that did not always produce them) when a gentleman riding in his chair invited him to take a lift. Finding the Frenchman an agreeable companion, the gentleman invited him into his house for dinner. Devèze demurred, saying he had just been to the chamber of a sick friend.

"And where were you going in such a hurry?" asked his host. "To Bush Hill."

"The Devil you were!" exclaimed the gentleman. "I hope you have not been there lately?"

"Oh yes!" said the Frenchman. "I am Dr. Devoze, one of the physicians who attend the hospital."

A highwayman with a pistol could not have frightened the gentleman more, commented Charles Biddle, who told the story in his diary. "He soon got rid of the Doctor, and never afterwards invited a stranger to ride with him."

IV

This Jean Devèze, who thus abruptly entered American history in the lee of Stephen Girard, was a man of substantial learning and noble spirit, a man of whom Girard could justly be proud. Born in the Hautes Pyrénées in 1753, trained in medicine at Bordeaux, he went to Santo Domingo when he was twenty-two. There he contracted yellow fever, but survived; shortly he returned to Paris for three years' more study. In 1778 he was back in Santo Domingo, as chief surgeon for the national troops of the Northern Province at Cap François. At Le Cap he established his own hospital, administering it along with his military duties, treating the fever constantly. He caught the disease himself a second time, a second time survived.

In the carnage of June he had barely escaped with his life. Carrying a little money, he fled on the ill-fated Philadelphia brig *Mary*, twice captured by British privateers who, of course, seized all French property, including Devèze's. "It was only after having been plundered in the most barbarous way," Devèze wrote, "and in violation of all personal rights, that we were allowed to continue on our journey." He reached Philadelphia on August 7, just as the fever was beginning.

Now Devèze was French, and his whole medical training was in the French tradition. Strangely, this tradition was almost entirely unknown to Philadelphians, for though the city was a great medical center, it was a center of Edinburgh and London medicine. Cullen, Brown, Lettsom, and the other great British teachers were as little interesting to Devèze as were his Bordeaux and Paris teachers to the Philadelphia doctors. But to Girard, familiar with French medicine, with Santo Domingo, and with Devèze's reputation, his appointment at Bush Hill seemed obvious, his presence in the city a stroke of good fortune.

Histories of the plague have been written by American doctors and their descendants, intellectual and lineal. They have been protagonists of one or another of the theories that were splitting the College of Physicians asunder. Poor Devèze, with his calm good sense and extraordinary success at Bush Hill, has received little notice. He was an alien in an alien land. The fact that he saved lives where others failed could not overcome the suspicion in which he was held. Yet his work at the hospital was truly remarkable. Dr. Nassy, another French physician, visited Bush Hill early in October. He found Devèze "a happy choice," uniting to a feeling heart the knowledge necessary for his task. He praised the cleanliness and neatness of every room, the vigilance of the French "under-surgeons" and American nurses:

Without prodigality, there is nothing wasted in that hospital. The most valuable medicines, the most exquisite wines, the nicest and most suitable diet, in short, every thing is in abundance, and every thing is destined for the relief of those unhappy and devoted persons, whom the epidemic has struck with its fatal blow.

Nassy was fulsome in his praise of the humane and generous charity of those who had "in a short time, and at their own expence, fitted up this new asylum for suffering humanity," and he mentioned the "assiduity and zeal of the committee that superintend it"; but he saw, more clearly than most, that the real achievement at Bush Hill was the work of the French surgeon.

Devèze himself paid his associates warmhearted tributes. Not a little of the success they earned, he asserted, was due to the "harmony which perpetually subsisted between Dr. Duffield and myself." Mrs. Saville, the matron, he pronounced "a valuable woman," and of Girard he could not say enough:

> Oh! you who pretend to philanthropy, reflect upon the indefatigable Girard! take him for your model, and profit by his lessons; and you, citizens of Philadelphia, may the name of Girard be ever dear to you!—If you, like me, had witnessed his virtuous actions, his brows would have been long ago adorned with a civic crown.

Devèze barely mentioned Helm; it was his French-speaking patron and friend on whom he spent his praises. He described Girard forsaking his business at great loss, coming each day to the hospital, making his inspection, and then visiting the patients:

> . . . the unfortunate persons in the greatest danger were those who first attracted his attention. He approached them with that philanthropy that proceeds from the heart alone, and which must give the greater lustre to his generous conduct: he encouraged, took them by the hand, and himself administered the medicines I prescribed. I even saw one of the diseased, who having nauseated his medicine, discharged the contents of his stomach upon his benefactor. What did Girard then do?—entirely devoted to the public welfare, firm and immovable, and forgetting himself to think only of the sufferings of his fellow-creatures, whom he wished to succour; he wiped the patient's cloaths, comforted, and by the force of persuasion and patience, induced him to swallow the remedy. He did not stop here —before he quitted him to shew the same attention to another, he felt his feet and head, in order to judge the degree of heat, that he might take from or add to his coverings, according to the nature of the case; he arranged the bed, inspired him with courage, by renewing in him the hope that he should recover.—From him he went to another, that vomited offensive matter that would have disheartened any other than this wonderful man; then seeing one at a distance at the point of death, with the eyes and skin yellow, covered with black blood, that run from both mouth and nostrils, and feeling about with a bloody and tremulous hand for a vessel which he could not obtain; Girard ran to his assistance, gave him the vase, replaced him in his bed, which he set to rights, and only quitted him to shew the same attention to another. The hour of repast arrives—he is hungry, yet complains of the necessity he was under of recruiting his strength; ran, eat a morsel in haste, and re-appeared immediately, still more earnest, and full of zeal to pay over again the same

attention; and never quitted but when forced by the calls of nature to take some few hours of rest.

Devèze had better clinical opportunities than any doctor to observe the fever, and everything he saw supported the conclusions he had drawn before he left Cap François: conclusions exactly opposed to those of Rush, for Devèze believed that the disease was not contagious, and was to be treated with gentle medicines. His art as a physician was not to oppose, but to assist nature; he had harsh words for those who violated his precepts:

It is when nature is inactive, art should shew itself; but how difficult to seize the critical moment *when the physician should only remain a spectator, or that when he ought to act.* He is an excellent physician who has acquired that degree of knowledge—happy the mortal that possesses him.

The logical, orderly theories and systems among which Rush roamed were no concern of the Frenchman's:

Being in the habit of seeing the diseased, and to observe nature, can alone guide the practitioner, and render medicine a really useful science, but any one who, seduced by the brilliancy of a system, will force nature by the rules of the method he has adopted, he, I say, is a scourge more fatal to the human kind than the plague itself would be.

Anyone who would force nature—Devèze here took his stand on Dr. Rush.

Many of the patients, he pointed out, came to Bush Hill only in the last extremities of disease, and many of them had received "very fatal medicines"—Dr. Rush's great purges of calomel, jalap, or gamboge. Medicines often killed, where illness could have been cured, Devèze boldly asserted.

He bled, under certain conditions, but in small quantities, in order to preserve the patients' strength. He opposed the copious and hasty bloodlettings of Rush, which he regarded as "mortal."

If his methods were not satisfactory in any one case, "I was not obstinate in continuing their use; I changed alternately from one to the other, till I found which best moderated and agreed with the immediate state of the solids." While Rush used the same cure in all cases, moving toward the position that all diseases were one disease, Devèze thought it wrong to believe that

what succeeded well in one case, would have the same success in all others, though they appeared alike; because often an infinite number of hidden circumstances produced a change in the animal economy. I have seen a remedy that has cured one, do no good to a second, and hurt a third. The diversity of effects proceeding from the same cause will always prevent specifics from becoming remedies generally; which means that medicine will never be as certain a science as experimental physics.

To Devèze the fact that he, Girard, Helm, many nurses and apothecaries, and the French soldiers later at Bush Hill, all remained uninfected, proved beyond any doubt that the disease was not contagious. There were two kinds of contagion, he wrote: that carried "by an efflux of miasmata spread through the air," and that arising from bodily contact. The staff of Bush Hill were continually exposed to both, with only three cases: Mrs. Saville, who recovered, and two nurses who died, one of them being "often disguised by liquor."

The lively doctor omitted no opportunity to learn everything he could. Of the 807 cases he and Duffield treated, he described seventeen in detail, and as often as he could he performed autopsies. "I opened a great number of bodies, and consequently was under the necessity of dipping my hands in the black and corrupted blood that proceeded from their mortified entrails, and breathed the infected vapours that exhaled from them." For Dr. Nassy he performed two post-mortems, one of a patient who had taken the drastic mercurial purges, the other treated in the mild French manner. Clearly, Nassy thought, the Rushite medicines were condemned: they wrought great havoc in the stomach and intestines, increasing the corrosive damage of the disease; they were proved wrong, not by theory, but by observed fact.

Bush Hill was the apparent, the inescapable refutation of Rush's enthusiastic claims, yet few would see the obvious truth. Devèze was a philosophic man. He accepted his lack of American popularity with good grace, understanding that he was a foreigner among proud and exclusive professional men. Later, as

his books on the fever appeared, he assumed the first rank
among continental authorities; but Rush ignored him entirely.
In all the writings of Benjamin Rush, the name of Jean Devèze
is not mentioned. The "American Sydenham" had some dubious
weapons in his armory.

Devèze was the least contentious of men, while Rush lived
life combatively; yet the Frenchman's reputation steadily grew
during the next century after the American's declined. Devèze's
*An Enquiry into, and Observations upon the Causes and Effects
of the Epidemic Disease Which Raged in Philadelphia from the
Month of August till towards the Middle of December 1793*
appeared in English and French texts in Philadelphia in 1794.
Ten years later, having returned to Paris, he received the degree of Doctor of Medicine for a revision of the *Enquiry,* called
Dissertation sur la Fièvre Jaune, and before his death (about
1826) he wrote four more volumes, widely circulated in Europe.
By 1854 Devèze was described, even by a Philadelphia writer,
as the highest authority on the yellow fever.

The Committee had received a greater aid than it realized, or
ever appreciated, when the quiet Santo Domingan appeared
before them.

v

Medical administration was the managers' only political problem, the only one on which they had a difference with the Committee. In everything else, the Committee adhered to its resolution vesting entire direction of Bush Hill in Girard and Helm.
Those two were not idle while the doctors' problems were being
settled. Helm found a spring in the vicinity and had the pumps
fixed, which brought water supply above normal. He and Girard
agreed that there should be some place to put convalescents apart
from the rest of the sick, and for this purpose began converting
the large stone barn behind the mansion. Committeeman Israel
Israel sent workmen to remove the hay and other things stored
there, and soon the barn was divided into three apartments—
one for the resident doctors and apothecaries, one for forty men

convalescents, one for fifty-seven women. This enabled the managers to report that they could receive and care for a much larger number of patients than under the previous system. By September 24, so rapidly had the Committee worked, and the hired carpenters, that Girard was able to say that all the sick were on bedsteads, with proper bedding, the rooms all numbered, and "the whole house is in regular order."

It was not long, however, before the number of patients outran facilities, even under the new system. As the death rate over the city increased, people were again laid on floors and in the halls. On October 2 the managers reported overcrowding, and the Committee at once ordered them and another member, Thomas Savery, to be in charge of building a new frame house sixty feet long by eighteen feet deep.

It went up in record time, a building complete with chimneys, having three rooms on the ground floor—one for the nurses and two containing seventeen beds each for the sick—and a loft with forty beds for convalescents. By October 6 William Hamilton, the carpenter, was discharged as no longer needed.

In one half of the old house, next to the mansion—that house which it had originally been intended to seize for the hospital—the tenant Thomas Boyles still lived (he must have viewed with dismay the fearful activity about a Bush Hill now unfamiliar to him), in the other half lived the cooks for the hospital; one cellar was occupied by the steward and clerk, the other was used for storing provisions. Some distance to the west of the mansion a frame building was hastily erected to store empty coffins and serve as a morgue where the dead could be laid before burial.

Advertisements for nurses and attendants produced few applicants, but some, attracted by motives of goodness or by the "generous wages," came to the Committee and offered their services. The managers were authorized to discharge the disorderly persons who had given the lazaretto such a foul name; on September 17 they reported they had hired nine female nurses and ten male attendants. On that day came Mrs. Mary Saville to the Committee, volunteering to act as assistant matron. A sober, clever, experienced woman, Mrs. Saville was engaged at $3 a day, and commenced "services . . . above all price." This invaluable female became head matron, and earned a gratitude almost equal to that paid Devèze, Girard, and Helm. The Committee ultimately resolved that she had "performed her duties with great propriety and fidelity," commended her unremitting care of the sick and her sympathetic and maternal attention to the afflicted.

The help changed from time to time as attendants died, fell ill, ran off, or were fired; but the general picture stabilized before the end of the month. The apothecary August Joseph Liber (or Libre) received $4 a day; so did Daniel Nicholas Morrice, Joseph Guizard, and one Muliner (or Mulnier)—these were French empirics and apothecaries whom Devèze brought in. They were casually referred to as "the resident doctors" or "the physicians" though they worked under Devèze and Duffield and were clearly not qualified practitioners of physic. One of them was charged with the distribution of food. At eleven o'clock he gave every patient broth with rice, bread, boiled beef, veal, mutton, and chicken, or lighter food if their case required it; at six o'clock he passed out broth, rice, and boiled prunes. With their meals the sick were given porter or claret and water, and throughout the day they took centaury tea and boiled lemonade.

A steward, Frederick Foy, and two waiters, Joseph Beaubrum and Jacob Decombe, one of whom was a barber and shaved the patients, and one of the two cooks, John Varrer (the other was Mistress Jane Wilson), completed the roll of the French staff. Bush Hill was run largely by the refugees—its head doctor, its four "physicians" or apothecaries, its steward, barber, and waiters all chattered in French among themselves and with the bilingual manager. Philadelphia was receiving in this one enterprise far more than just return for its summer's charities. Frenchmen and Santo Domingans were bringing a good order and cleanliness which native leadership had been unable to produce.

Few of the patients, however, and none of the nurses, were French. Peter Rose and his wife were first nurses, Peter receiving $24 a month until both unaccountably disappeared from the record. The rest—Irish, English, and unidentifiable—received a dollar a day at first, later $3 a week. Besides the nurses there were washerwomen and laborers and the various artisans hired by the Committee, and some recovered patients who stayed on at Bush Hill as nurses. Two of the last, John Johnson and Priscilla Hicks, came into the city on September 23 to be married, and returned to their work at the hospital; on November 5 one Nassy, a Portuguese mulatto employed as a nurse, married Hannah Smith, "a bouncing German girl," who worked beside him.

In supplies the Committee served the managers efficiently. Supplies involved no controversy over theories or men. Any request Girard and Helm made was immediately fulfilled, or at least ordered to be fulfilled. So far as the Committee sitting at City Hall could get what the hospital needed, they did: when the managers report "a number of articles wanting," a list is made and the materials ordered to be sent out early tomorrow; a "large supply of sheets, blankets &c being immediately necessary," Thomas Wistar and Henry Deforest are requested "to take their instructions from the managers and procure every necessary that may be required for the use of the sick at the Hospital." The managers announce "a great want of the herb centaury," and the Committee prints four hundred handbills asking for a supply.

In nothing did the new order at the hospital so clearly express itself as in the keeping of records. Before Girard and Helm took charge, apparently no memoranda had been made of admissions, cures, deaths, and dismissals. The new managers began at once, however, to enroll cases and their outcome. Alphabetically in a big ledger they entered names, dates, and results. Admitted September 18, John Andre died on the twenty-fifth. Admitted on September 18, Dolly Benjamin was convalescent by October 9:

Sept. 23.	Christy, Andrew.	Sept. 28, Dead
Sept. 23.	Calleghan, Martha.	Sept. 25, Dead
Sept. 23.	Collin, Julian.	Octo. 1, Dead
Sept. 23.	Correll, Patrick.	Convalescent
Sept. 23.	Conrads, Elizabeth	Convalescent
Sept. 23.	Christy, Mary.	Sept. 30, Dead
Sept. 23.	Creery, Hannah.	Discharged

Far too many entries had the dismal note "Dead" after the name. Even under the new system, half the patients were lost. Part of the reason for this was that many patients did not come to Bush Hill until they were far advanced in disease. Doctors Cathrall, Leib, and Physick had memorialized the Committee on this point, asking them

to prevail upon our fellow citizens to send those who are designed for the Hospital, as early as possible after they take the disorder; as the chance of recovery in case of an immediate removal is very flattering, but that the contrary must be expected to be the consequence of delay.

This was published in the newspapers in the middle of September, but it had little effect, for people still dreaded the hospital as a grave. The new managers continually faced the same problem of receiving patients only after they were in a hopeless condition. On the twenty-first they asked the Committee once again to persuade people to come as soon as they knew themselves to be infected: "many have deferred it so long, that they have died on their way, and most who die at the Hospital, expire within two days after their admission."

Secretary Caleb Lownes published another address to citizens; but the next week Dr. Duffield still had to report that "several who were admitted yesterday were in the last stages of the disorder, that in general the persons who die are those who have not been there above two or three days . . ." As daily death rates mounted, the managers waxed more urgent in their representations. Eighteen patients died within twenty-four hours on October 4, "the greater part of them having been sent out within a few days last past." One had died in the cart on the way. The general prospect was favorable, the managers said, "and could the citizens be prevailed upon to go out as soon as they are attacked by the disorder, the lives of many might be preserved." On October 5 eight were buried, five of whom had been received less than a day before.

This problem of timely admissions was never solved, even though public confidence in Bush Hill rose as the work of the managers progressed. Some improvement was noted, however, even by Dr. William Annan, a Rushite. Much later, when Rush did a bit of enquiring about the hospital, Dr. Annan wrote him that early reports of its inadequate staff and care at Bush Hill acted powerfully upon the sick poor, persuading them to conceal their indisposition as long as possible. This continued to be true, Annan observed, until "the latter end of September," when a report was circulated that the hospital had enough nurses and bedding:

A report was propagated at the same time that the Great French Physicians Girard and Deveze had discovered the nature of the disease and method of cure; Without commenting on the validity of the report I can inform You that it had the desired effect. For no sooner was a Person affected with a headache or oppression about the Praecordia than he became anxious to be removed to Bushhill Hospital.

Frequently Annan had to examine patients with other diseases who applied to go to the lazaretto. His information was scarcely satisfying to Rush, whose whole medical theory and method Bush Hill so dramatically impeached. Rush publicly admitted that the institution, after the Committee took it in charge, "was well regulated and governed with the order and cleanliness of an old and established hospital." In his published essays he added only the unvarnished and obliquely worded observation, "An American and French physician had the exclusive medical care of it after the 22d of September," though privately he had more to say.

Dr. George Logan of Stenton visited Bush Hill at the Committee's request and handed in a report which Caleb Lownes sent to Brown's *Gazette,* praising the whole arrangement of the hospital. He had found everything perfectly clean, no offensive smell, the sick well accommodated and tenderly cared for "by citizens Girard and Helm, who, on this occasion, merit in a high degree, the thanks of their fellow citizens." He had followed the physicians on their rounds, Logan wrote, and found them attentive, rational, and correct. He also urged sending the sick there as soon as possible.

The real character of the managers' days was shaped not by these administrative details and staff problems, important as they were, but by the pitiable realities around them. What gave Bush Hill its meaning and fashioned the human experience Girard and Helm were having was the presence of fivescore of the sick, dying, and dead on any one day. The spectacle was indescribable. Human life was not cheap at the hospital, yet it was spent with tragic prodigality. For the dying, Girard acted as confessor and chaplain, comforter and attorney. Robert Tait of Kentucky, merchant, took the fever while on a visit to the city. His landlord, the tavern keeper Barnabas McShane, hurried him out to Bush Hill where he gasped away his life as Girard, a notary public, took down his last will and testament. To his brother, "William Tait, of the Western Country," he left all he had on him when he died, a poor fortune in pocket which Girard gathered and delivered to the Committee. After Captain Burrows died, the managers likewise sent his property in, and later in the month collected and labeled "sundry small packages" containing the effects of deceased patients, handing them to Henry Deforest to be held by him until claimed. Such entries continued on the Committee's books:

The managers Report, Colonel Perry and William Grenville are both dead, they now deposit sundry articles which were the property of the former in the hands of the committee, as per list, to be held for the use of his daughter and heirs when they may appear, the will of the latter was handed to the committee who he hath appointed his executors.

For Girard, time stood still these endless days at Bush Hill. His private business was entirely neglected: "I have to devote myself to the public welfare," he told one client, "and whenever I have a moment to spare I spend it in looking after your interests." The hospital absorbed all his energies, but even when he went home he found the fever still the dominant fact in his life. "We are in a deplorable condition," he wrote a correspondent. "It is now the 30th of September. Poor Mr. Delmas who came here in the brig *La Couronne* died yesterday at 10 o'clock in the evening after three days of fever. I do not know when our misfortunes will end."

A young Irishman, Peter Seguin, arrived in the city from one of Girard's merchant-house correspondents at Bordeaux, and on Wednesday, October 2, dined with Girard in his home. He joined the young clerks in their amusements, and moved in with the family, doing odd jobs in the warehouse until he could get a vessel to Baltimore. On October 10 he caught the fever. "I am his doctor," Girard wrote, "and although he is constantly delirious, I hope that the treatment, a *grand lavage,* with the strength of his constitution will enable him to go to you on the *Abigail.*" The poor young man grew worse, however, and Devèze was called. Girard, returning from his work at the hospital, would sit with his young Irish friend until the dawn. In spite of tender care and Devèze's plasters, poor Seguin died. Girard buried him in the Catholic cemetery.

The improved and efficient hospital did not stop the disease; no one had expected it would. But it did do a great deal to stop the panic. Girard and Helm constructed a clean and orderly place which people grew eventually no longer to fear. Carey observed that in a few weeks people began to apply for admission, and indeed so many applied who had diseases other than the fever that it finally became necessary to require a certificate from a physician that he was suffering from the prevailing disease before a patient would be accepted.

For the two managers Philadelphians had endless encomiums. "If an ancient Roman, who saved the life of one citizen, at the risque of his own, was crowned with a civic wreath, what rewards do these men deserve? who were instrumental in saving the lives of many!" asked the anonymous author of *An Account of . . . the Malignant Fever*. "They gave up their own to help the helpless. . . ."

The Committee

SEPTEMBER 15–OCTOBER 10

A number of citizens however, with a courage that will always do them honor, formed themselves into a Committee headed by the Mayor; borrowed money on credit of future subscriptions; established an hospital, about a mile from town, for the poor; procured carriages to convey the sick to it; sat daily at the City Hall to receive applications and administer relief . . .

—SAMUEL AND MIERS FISHER
Circular, November 1793

WHILE the managers were achieving their reforms at Bush Hill, and giving the city hope thereby, the picture downtown was going from very bad to much worse. Fully half the inhabitants had fled, some thought; certainly the number was very large, yet "the malignant action of the disease increased, so that those who were in health one day were buried the next."

So wrote the merchant Samuel Breck, and he added:

The burning fever occasioned paroxysms of rage which drove the patient naked from his bed to the street, and in some instances to the river, where he was drowned. Insanity was often the last stage of its horrors.

Breck (himself safe in the country) told of a householder in whose stable lay a stranger racked with fever. The householder went to City Hall to see the Committee about having him removed. The scene at City Hall was turbulent and strange.

173

The attendants on the dead stood on the pavement in considerable numbers soliciting jobs, and until employed they were occupied in feeding their horses out of the coffins which they had provided in anticipation of their daily wants. These speculators were useful, and, albeit with little show of feeling, contributed greatly to lessen, by competition, the charges of interment.

Making his way through this grisly throng, the householder finally reached the room in which the Committee sat, and obtained from them "the services of a quack doctor, none other being in attendance." The empiric came, looked at the patient, pronounced him dying, and appointed an hour when he would send the coffin. He proved an accurate guesser.

There was nothing orderly or dignified in the surroundings of City Hall these days. Indeed, the place was a confusion of frantic activity and patient waiting, in which there was really more system than appeared, for the Mayor's Committee was contributing its share to the revival of courage in the city. Courage, like panic, is contagious. The committeemen set examples of resolute determination which no one failed to see, and many followed.

The Committee of citizens, formed on that Saturday, September 14, "to transact the whole of the business relative to the sick," soon found the whole of that business to be the whole business of the city. Before a week had passed, Philadelphia was being ruled by its new, determined, extralegal little legislature. Of all the brands of heroism produced in the stricken city that fall, not the least admirable was the brand displayed by the handful of "benevolent citizens" who gathered around the Mayor.

Handful it was. Though twenty-six volunteers made up the original Committee (and two joined later) only half of them proved actually effective. Four of the benevolent citizens disappeared entirely after the organizing meeting on the fourteenth. Others, having worked a while, decided to leave example to their colleagues and fled to the safer country. Girard and Helm were entirely occupied with Bush Hill. And death took its toll: four of the most active members died at the very height of the plague.

After death had removed its share, and fear, what the Mayor had left was a small company of devoted citizens, a dozen of them. Forty-six days, from September 16 to October 31, they came to his office, forty-six times called the roll. They sat all day, every day, Sundays too; they assumed the tasks of government.

They were a strangely assorted lot. Some of them the Mayor had never met before. Others it would certainly never have occurred to him to appoint, had the choice been his to make. But that was the great thing about the Committee—they had chosen themselves. Out of the desperation of disease and death, out of the disorganization of community life, these men had emerged, self-selected, uncompelled. They were the irreducible minimum of leadership.

Curious what men a crisis uncovers. And what qualities it finds in them. Samuel Benge, umbrella maker, for example: he was just over from London. He owed Philadelphia nothing. Yet as soon as Mayor Clarkson called for volunteers, Benge walked across Chestnut Street and offered his services. Quietly this English shopkeeper began to work. He assumed the most opprobrious of all tasks—carrying the sick and burying the dead. And he was the only member of the Committee who had a perfect record of attendance, at all forty-six meetings.

Henry Deforest was only a cabinetmaker. He had counted for very little in the city's affairs. But now Henry Deforest was to become food administrator for the whole city in siege, and receiver of properties, a sort of quartermaster general. He attended forty-four of the forty-six Committee meetings.

And John Letchworth was a windsor-chair maker, James Sharswood and Thomas Savery were carpenters, James Kerr a coachmaker. From such artisans, mechanics, and small tradesmen came the new leaders—from, as Carey said, "the middle walks of life." Joseph Inskeep was a schoolmaster, James Swain a mechanic, Andrew Adgate—well, Adgate was one of the most curious people in all the city. He earned his living as a card maker, but he was Philadelphia's premier music master, founder of a free school of music called the Uranian Academy, organizer and director of great vocal concerts every year, still remembered for the Grand Concert of Sacred Music he conducted in 1786 for the benefit of the medical institutions of the city, the greatest aggregation of singers and musicians that had ever been gathered together in America. Every public occasion needed music, and Philadelphians always sent for Andrew Adgate and his choir. Now the bright little man appeared in a new role, moved by an impulse of goodness that was to cost his life.

They were conscientious and devoted, these committeemen. To make roll call every day was a matter of pride with them, and when they had to be away they made a point of explaining their absence. For example, Thomas Harrison, cobbler and currier, a pious Quaker—Harrison had no sooner started his work on the Committee than his son fell ill. Several of his family had already died. A doctor told him to take his son out to the country. It was his only hope. Friend Harrison asked the Committee for leave before he went up to Bristol.

At Bristol some Quakers from the city saw him. "He is a lively active benevolent man," one of them wrote, "but his fine spirits are gone, and he could scarcely speak without tears."

And there was John Connelly. Connelly attended Committee regularly for a while, then was a long time absent. When he next turned up at City Hall he explained to the other members that his wife and family had been ill, and nursing them had taken all his time. The Committee, proud of its conscientiousness, still had no desire to condemn absent members. They spread upon their minutes the note that Connelly had been "repeatedly attacked" by the fever, "and when able to be abroad was constantly employed in visiting the sick whose destitute situation rendered such friendly offices more than usually necessary."

Catholic Mathew Carey went even further in explaining Connelly's absences. Connelly, he wrote, "spent hours beside the sick, when their own wives and children had abandoned them. Twice did he catch the disorder—twice was he on the brink of the grave, which was yawning to receive him—yet, unappalled by the imminent danger he had escaped, he again returned to the charge."

Those who never left, even when their own families were sick, needed no justifications or excuses. Volunteers, they served with a faithfulness no authority could have compelled, in horrors which the wise, the rich, the sensible had fled.

A heavy burden fell on Caleb Lownes, the secretary. If it was Matthew Clarkson's part to organize, administer, inspirit the Committee, it was Lownes's to execute orders, to translate resolutions into action. Lownes was an iron merchant, another "drawn from the middle walks of life." The city knew little of him. His only public exercise had been a pamphlet describing the Walnut Street Prison. Now Lownes's desk became the administrative nerve center of the city. Only twice in the forty-six days was he missing from it.

Clarkson organized and presided, Lownes recorded and administered, but the actual legwork devolved upon other committeemen, upon none more frequently than the busy Israel Israel. He was the field officer of this little command.

Reserved, handsome, swarthy, foreign-looking, Israel Israel was forty-seven in 1793, and unlike most of his colleagues was a conspicuous figure in the city. Hardie listed him in the *Directory* as "innkeeper and livery stabler, 89, Chestnut St." Sixty years after his death a Masonic orator would describe him as "an Israelite in whom there was no guile." Both descriptions were misleading. There was in Israel Israel all the guile of a local politician; he had not a drop of Jewish blood; and he was a man of substance whose inn and livery stable were only minor interests.

Actually, Israel was a third-generation Philadelphian. His father was of Dutch Protestant descent, his mother a Scotch-Irish Paxton; he was an Episcopalian. As a young man he had gone to Barbados and made a fortune. He returned, married Hannah Erwin, engaged in petty politics, and now proved himself a noble, conscientious civic being. Ultimately he would become High Sheriff of Philadelphia and Masonic Grand Master. Now what most Philadelphians knew of him was a romantic hero-legend of the Revolutionary War.

Member of the Committee of Safety, Israel had found himself in Wilmington after the battle of the Brandywine, and when Howe occupied Philadelphia, Israel was concerned over the fate of his father and mother. He walked from Wilmington to Philadelphia. He encountered a Tory friend en route who gave him the British password. At his parents' home Israel found British soldiers quartered, but nevertheless arranged a secret rendezvous with his brother Joseph, of the Continental army. After Joseph, the British raised a hue and cry; so Israel trudged back to Wilmington, there to be informed against by the same Tory who had passed him through the British lines. Imprisoned on the frigate *Roebuck* lying in the bay just off his own Delaware farm, Israel suffered torments physical and mental. Learning that he owned cattle, the British officers ordered his herd seized. But his young bride Hannah, then only nineteen, with the aid of a farm boy drove away the cows and saved them for Washington's army. Meanwhile Israel secured his release by giving the Masonic sign to his captors.

Israel was a man of wealth, though pro-French and anti-Federalist. He could easily have fled to Delaware, or up the river. Instead, he went about the city every day, poked his shapely nose into everything, attended Committee more than forty times.

Also wealthy was Samuel Wetherill, the Committee's vice-president. Wetherill was a prosperous manufacturing druggist and dealer in painters' colors. His presence gave the Committee prestige. But after attending four times the first week, Mr. Wetherill was seen no more, except once: on October 4 he came to tell the Committee of illness and deaths in his family, of his stricken neighbors, of the many calls upon him. He reported that most of the apothecary shops were closed, that he had to make and distribute medicines and care for his sick ones. He resigned.

More faithful was the merchant Thomas Wistar, treasurer, brother to Dr. Caspar Wistar. He placed all his personal credit behind the financing of the Committee. He attended every day for twenty-nine meetings, until October 17. Then he fell ill, and was taken out to Germantown; his financial duties were assumed by others.

Wetherill could have spared Clarkson many tasks. His credit alone would have solved problems. And Wistar's illness was a serious loss. The rich and well-born, the mercantile gentry, the Federalists, were not carrying their share of the load. But the Mayor was finding his new friends—the artisans, shopkeepers, small tradesmen—equal to every demand upon them. It was amazing, how the core of his Committee proved to be of these humble persons. The fever was now the common people's problem, and the common people had produced their own leaders. Conservative, well-to-do Matthew Clarkson found strange companions in the plague.

But they were the right companions—Israel, Benge, Kerr, Deforest, Adgate, the others—for they were doing the work required. And the Mayor found three old friends on his Committee—three friends that almost made up for the loss of Wetherill. Daniel Offley was a noted Quaker preacher; he was also a leading merchant with a warehouse at the Arch Street Wharf. Offley joined the group at the beginning of the second week. Mathew Carey, the publisher (Clarkson was one of his backers), returned to town on October 8 and began to work with true Irish energy on the Committee's poor relief. And the Mayor could take heart every day as he saw Jonathan Dickinson Sergeant come into his chambers. Sergeant was politically radical, but he was a fine lawyer, trustee of the University, son-in-law to Dr. Rittenhouse, former attorney-general of the commonwealth.

With Dr. Hutchinson, Dr. Michael Leib, the Governor's secretary Dallas, the merchant Coates, the political Israel Israel, and the radical Charles Biddle, Sergeant had organized in May the Democratic Society. It was the heart of pro-French, Republican sentiment, the focus of animosity against Hamilton, Washington, and Federalism generally. Sergeant and his friends had feted Genêt. They had set new revolutionary machinery in motion. Sergeant was a man of birth and position embracing the popular cause. Now he proved himself an even rarer being—a friend of the common man in theory who could live with common men in practice, joyously serve them, and share their lot.

While the Federal gentry fled, Mayor Clarkson received his real help from artisans, radicals, revolutionaries, from those whom the gentry regarded as dangerous. There was a lesson here, somewhere.

II

September was no time for politics, however, or October. These were days only for work. If the Committee was to mean anything, it required money. Caleb Lownes, Thomas Wistar, and Thomas Harrison had signed personal notes for the first $1,500 loan from the Bank of North America. The Committee agreed that a public subscription would be filled later, and bank president John Nixon offered the money without interest. Treasurer Wistar used this fund to purchase all that was needed for Bush Hill, to hire laborers, pay carriers, even to pay Absalom Jones and Richard Allen for burying the dead. The Committee also voted to give or lend money to poverty-stricken families with the disease. The $1,500 was not going to last very long.

Particularly, it was not going to last if the committeemen expanded their services. Yet everything the members did required money, and they were forever finding new burdens to assume. As soon as Girard and Helm took over Bush Hill, the rest of the members began to parcel out tasks among themselves. Each had talents or experience that determined what his work should be. Thomas Wistar, for example, with his knowledge of banking and commerce, handled all financial details. He signed vouchers and checks; he also received the gifts of cash that began coming in at once from individuals and merchant houses.

And to procure carriages, carts, wagons, and hearses, to

manage the whole matter of transport for doctors, patients, and dead, the coachmaker James Kerr, the windsor-chair maker John Letchworth, were perfectly fitted. One by one special jobs were assigned. The cabinetmaker Henry Deforest took charge of procuring coffins. He also became custodian of the property of the dead taken from their pockets when they were put in coffins, later of all property personal and real of which they died possessed.

The dead who seemed not to belong to anyone had to be buried, the sick without family or friends had to be taken to Bush Hill. Samuel Benge accepted these duties. He was a sub-committee of one, this British umbrella man. He came to be called Superintendent of Burials and Removals. Frequently he had to transport the sick himself, yet he was always at City Hall for roll call. Benge took a few of Anderson's Pills each day and a little sweet oil every evening. He escaped infection.

Benge's sad routine was to hand Secretary Lownes a list of each day's dead, and receive back orders for burial. It was a regular part of the daily agenda for Lownes to record the number of burials the managers reported at Bush Hill, and the number buried by Benge at public expense from the rest of the city. Thus, on September 18 the managers reported eight deaths, Lownes added six more from Benge's figures. On October 4 eighteen died at Bush Hill, fourteen were buried by Benge. On October 12 Bush Hill lost twenty-seven, the city twenty-nine. These were the pauper victims, those to whom the African Society's carriers were not called. The Committee's every session ended with the grim totals noted in Lownes's minutes.

Benge hired a poor man named Thomas Wilkinson as carter, to remove the sick poor by day and bury the dead by night. Wilkinson worked steadily through the whole pestilence, with loyal perseverance. The stink of his cart was insupportable. Frequently he was seen to vomit as he returned from duty. Once, hoisting into his wagon the corpse of a woman several days dead, he was covered with putrid blood. Yet Wilkinson lasted till November 4 before he caught the disease.

Going about the town, committeemen found scores of tasks
to do, scores of needs to report. A member entered a Santo
Domingan's lodgings and discovered both husband and wife
dead, twin babies helpless. Two committeemen investigated,
collected all the property, found a home for the children. There
were problems like this every day; they were solved by rule of
thumb.

Just what powers should be assumed by the Committee, and
what avoided, no one quite knew, so the members did anything
that seemed necessary. When a citizen complained of the route
taken by carters in removing the dead from Bush Hill, it was
easy to fix a new one: down Broad Street to Walnut and thence
to Potter's Field. But when someone proposed they should care
for the children wandering homeless and orphaned in the streets,
committeemen seriously questioned whether this fell within the
scope of "business relative to the sick."

The children were starving, however, and had no place to go.
They were being "shunned as a pestilence," Carey said, because
their parents had died of fever. One little group of orphans from
a well-to-do family was found huddled around a blacksmith's
forge, hungry, dirty, and afraid.

This was the Committee's first week; whatever they did
would set a precedent. But after some discussion, the Committee agreed that these children, as well as "sufferers of other
descriptions," deserved their attention. Israel Israel, James
Kerr, and Thomas Harrison were appointed to find a house for
·the orphans and see to their support.

Next day Israel reported they had obtained a house. He was
thereupon asked to collect the children, "see that they are
properly accommodated and treated," and to remove any with
fever to the hospital.

This was September 19. The house chosen was William
Ralston's in Fifth Street, which Israel obtained by paying one
quarter's rent (£12). There he, Kerr, and Harrison took thirteen children, and engaged Mistress Mary Parvin as matron.
Thirteen children was a large order for the good lady, but soon

others began to come her way, duly admitted on the Committee's authority. After three weeks had passed, fourteen more had come, sometimes as many as five from one family. And Lownes kept a careful record of each one:

Owen McGarvey and Henry Spence were admitted into the Orphan house, McGarvey's father and mother both died at the Hospital at Bush Hill. . . .
Lott Davis, John Miller, Mary Smith, Ann Maria Anthony and three children of Forbes Newton were sent to the orphan house. . . .

Sometimes children from one family would be brought in, and days later their brothers and sisters would be found wandering in the streets.

Once started with the orphan problem, the Committee could not let it go; but it was a big job, second only to Bush Hill in scope and expense. Just as the managers formed a subcommittee for the hospital and to Samuel Benge was left the problem of removals and burials, so Israel, Kerr, and Harrison became the Orphan Committee, in charge of the asylum. Thomas Harrison, however, left town just as the work began, so the tasks of organizing, staffing, supervising, and supplying the orphan house fell on James Kerr and the ubiquitous Israel Israel. On September 22 the Quaker minister Daniel Offley came to City Hall. He asked to be permitted to help in the service of the poor, so he was added to the Orphan Committee in Harrison's place.

By September 25 the children were housed and cared for, but they needed clothes. Everyone with spare children's things was asked to send them to City Hall. By the thirtieth the Ralston house was straining at the beam-ends, so Israel, Kerr, and Offley looked about for "a more commodious and airy situation." There were certainly plenty of empty houses all around, but the Committee's gaze lighted at once on the building at Sixth and Walnut, across from the prison on one side and State House Yard on the other, "the house lately made use of for and known by the name of the Loganian Library." This pleasant little structure had been designed and built by James Logan in 1745, and housed his books until they had been moved just a few months past to the

front room of the Library Company's new building in Fifth
Street. It had high ceilings and large rooms; it was now, the
Orphan Committee learned, the property of John Swanwick. To
him on September 30 Israel Israel went a-begging.

Swanwick, a prosperous merchant, told Israel he had rented
the building to one of the French fireworks makers, a man
named André Varinot, but he would at once try to secure its
release. He would even himself pay for any alterations "to
render it convenient and suitable for the purpose designed."
Before the day was over, the building was transferred, though
the tenant later (like William Hamilton of Bush Hill) had
some questions to ask. André Varinot wrote the Committee
saying he had from motives of benevolence submitted to the
demands upon him, but pointed out that he had paid $48 for
half a year's rent, had repaired a window and closet in the
garret, had been forced to give up an excellent situation for his
business in favor of a poor one, and he still had to pay rent on
the new house Swanwick had found for him. Would the committee indemnify him for his rent and pay him for the rent and
the repairs?

The Committee was too busy to answer, and they had already
moved in. On October 1 Israel, Kerr, and Offley reported they
had "this day taken possession of the house lately the Loganian
Library for an orphan house."

More children were admitted, and the whole enterprise became a large one in its new quarters, requiring three men and
seven women to assist the matron, as well as a number of wet
nurses who received children in their own homes. Dr. Samuel
Duffield (brother of Benjamin at Bush Hill) was engaged to
visit the house regularly to give medical aid. Israel, Kerr, and
Offley could not carry the whole of this burden themselves, so
on October 3 the Committee added James Sharswood and John
Letchworth to the Orphan Committee, to supervise the house
and the wet nurses' homes, to gather more children, to keep the
records. Records were particularly difficult to keep, for some
of the children could not be identified. Daily reports were ren-

dered just as at Bush Hill: "Christiana and Elinor Wossem, Willie, Thomas and Ann Cresswell; Rachel Obercow and two children of the name of Brayley" were admitted on October 4; a mulatto child on the fifth, four Sweeneys and Catherine Summers on the sixth, five Eastwicks and half a dozen others on the seventh, and as the adult death rate mounted an ever greater number each day. Ultimately, Mayor Clarkson was to report that 192 "helpless innocents" came under the Committee's care, of whom 94 were reclaimed by their "friends," 27 died, 71 remained public charges.

At any time, there would be three to four dozen of the children "out at nurse." This made the problem of supervision particularly difficult and added to the hazards of the Orphan Committee in inspecting. Wet nurses lived in tiny houses, in close, airless streets. As Daniel Offley went about on his rounds visiting nurses, collecting children who had lost both parents, or had lost one and the other was sick, he himself contracted the disease. On October 3 he failed to appear at City Hall. He lay at home, cared for by a Negro nurse, desperately ill but apparently convalescing. Then one night his nurse fell asleep. Offley had neither drink nor food for many hours. On October 12 he died.

The Library was soon outgrown. Washing sheds and other outbuildings were erected; finally a room 30 by 14 feet, nearly half as large as the original building, was added. So many children came with property tied in handkerchiefs, or were legally entitled to some inheritance, that Israel Israel arranged for a systematic public guardianship. The plight of the innocents was everywhere appealing. Many donations came in earmarked "for the use of the orphans" or for "a distressed family of children." This income was of great help to the Committee in its financial struggle. A curious problem arose when some of the older children turned out to be bound boys. They were returned to their masters as soon as they could be, but when merchants, among them the printer Robert Aitken, applied to take some of the children as apprentices, the Committee firmly refused. Aitken was told "that none of these children can be disposed of upon this principle."

The Orphan Committee, like the managers, became a permanent part of the Committee and its work. Israel, Kerr, Sharswood, and Letchworth, among their other duties, were continually busy overseeing the hospice. Their achievement compared significantly with Bush Hill: ultimately the total cost at the orphan house came to about $20 per child; at Bush Hill it was only $11 per patient. Mortality at Bush Hill was about fifty per cent; among the children (entirely from causes other than fever) it was about fifteen per cent.

III

The Orphan Committee was only one of the activities of the men who met daily in the council chamber at City Hall. A host of other tasks confronted them, tasks incident to the operation of a large city. A blind man needed his accustomed charitable allowance as he departed to visit friends in the country; the Committee voted him a dollar a week for three weeks. The Guardians of the Poor of the Northern Liberties, who stayed at their posts taking up the sick and burying the dead, needed a horse and cart; the Committee agreed to supply them. But when a landlord requested the Committee to pay the arrears of his tenants' rents, he received a cold refusal.

Someone complained that coffinmakers were careless, were not applying enough pitch to their boxes. Foul fluids from bodies could be seen oozing through the boards. The Committee rebuked the crafters and enjoined them to be more careful in the future. "Many injurious reports" were circulated that the dead were thrown indiscriminately into trenches in Potter's Field, with no coffins. Joseph Ogden, the sexton of Potter's Field, was asked to come to City Hall and account for his work. Ogden convinced the Committee that such reports were groundless, and asked them to inspect the graveyard and clear his character. Israel Israel and James Sharswood, their faces covered, viewed the ground and came back announcing all was well, the rumors false, the burials "proper and safe." Secretary Lownes sent a letter to Brown's paper to that effect.

Each member was busy with similar short-run tasks while at the same time engaged in more permanent assignments. "Persons unknown" who died at Bush Hill had to be identified, their property held by Henry Deforest along with all the rest of the unclaimed goods he was receiving. Complaints of infected bedding not burned or buried were investigated by Thomas Savery. The demand for coffins far exceeded the supply, prices charged rose daily higher, the Committee directed Savery (himself a carpenter) to find out how many coffinmakers there were, and what they earned. Israel Israel was asked to see to the harvesting of grain on the Bush Hill farm and have it stacked. Rumors came in about improper management of burial grounds other than Potter's Field; Mathew Carey was appointed to investigate.

Back and forth through the dusty, saddened city the Committeemen went, on foot, on horse, or in carriages, doing what they could as individuals, reporting back to City Hall when they encountered something too big for their own efforts. It was a dangerous job. On September 30 the music master Andrew Adgate died; he had been sick five days. On October 5 Jonathan Dickinson Sergeant failed to attend; he died on the eighth. The schoolmaster Joseph Inskeep, who had won a brief fame throughout the city for kindness and bravery, died on October 16. These, with Daniel Offley, were the victims of their own benevolence. Inskeep had been, Carey averred, the foremost of the noble group:

To the sick and the forsaken has he devoted his hours, to relieve and comfort them in their tribulation, and his kind assistance was dealt out with equal freedom to an utter stranger as to his bosom friend. Numerous are the instances of men restored, by his kind cares and attention, to their families, from the very jaws of death. In various cases has he been obliged to put dead bodies into coffins, when the relations fled from the mournful office.

Yet when Inskeep and his wife both fell ill and sent for help to a neighboring family whom he had nursed, they were coldly refused any assistance.

The Mayor's constant presence made it possible for the Committee frequently to act with the color of legal authority, and they did not hesitate to do so. Elijah Weed, keeper of the prison, reported two prisoners "lately committed for slight offenses" were sick with the fever, and asked that they be released. The Committee agreed, so Clarkson ordered them discharged and sent to Bush Hill.

Moved by this incident, the Mayor walked across State House Yard to the prison to see for himself how it was faring. He inspected the whole establishment, peering with his crooked gaze into every corner. He found "health, industry, quietness and cleanliness prevailing there in a pleasing degree."

Warden Elijah Weed was not comfortable, however, for a number of French soldiers and sailors had been sent to his jail at Citizen Genêt's request, charged with no crime but held as deserters. Weed, and the Committee, too, wanted them removed, not only because they were possible carriers of the disease but for fear of riots against them should fever start in the prison. Twice Mayor Clarkson wrote Genêt, who had removed to New York; finally the Minister responded, referring Clarkson to "Secretary Bournonville" for the disposition of the deserters. But Secretary Bournonville had fled to the country, and could not be found for weeks. Meanwhile, the French deserters remained in the jail, a worrisome problem and a threat.

Warden Weed was useful to the Committee in many ways. When Caleb Lownes went about seeking beds for Bush Hill, Weed supplied them from his prison stores. Later he volunteered to take charge of all the farm produce and livestock sent from rural counties of Pennsylvania, Jersey, and Delaware, a service particularly useful to the Committee since they had no storage space of their own. Weed conducted the prison so well that no inmates contracted the fever. Repeated inspections pronounced it "clean, healthy and in good order." But the humane Weed, moving through the city on all sorts of volunteer work, caught the disease, and fell a victim to it. His death, and his daughter's, were the only fatalities at the Walnut Street Jail.

The three Guardians of the Poor—Wilson, Sansom, Tomkins —could no longer attend to their regular duties. They were wholly occupied with the business of finding, collecting, removing the sick and burying the dead, under the direction of Samuel Benge. But the poor, customarily public charges, had still to be cared for, whether or not they had the fever. The Committee was obliged to assume this work as well—to administer ordinary poor relief to the starving, homeless, and old. On September 20 a subcommittee of distribution was appointed, with Israel Israel as its head. It was directed "to receive applications from the poor, and administer such relief as their circumstances may render necessary and proper." This was taking over a state-government function, and it was enormously expensive. Yet poor relief was added to the already heavy burdens of Bush Hill, the orphan house, and the growing payroll for carters, workmen, and gravediggers. Israel's committee of distribution had to turn down many applicants and practice every economy. At the Committee's direction, they visited the Almshouse, to find out if that institution could accept any more paupers.

The managers of the Almshouse had resolved on September 9 that no more paupers be admitted, in an attempt to keep the fever out. All of the managers had fled town by the twentieth, however, and the steward frankly informed the Committee that there was plenty of room—the house could accommodate two hundred more inmates than it had. To send more there legally was impossible, in view of the managers' resolves. But Mayor Clarkson proceeded with little regard for legalities. He and Alderman Hilary Baker prepared blanks for admitting paupers to the Almshouse, "conformably to Law," as they said, in spite of the managers' regulation, and at once a pauper named Hugh Ferguson, "being recommended by Nicholas Waln and Doctor Park, as a suitable object," was sent to the institution.

The resources of the Almhouse thus opened, pressure was relieved. But financial problems were beginning to appear at every step in the Committee's way. On September 24, confronted with ever larger demands upon them, the Committee sent Thomas Wistar and Jonathan Dickinson Sergeant back to the Bank of North America for another loan. A new subscription was opened, and John Nixon "cheerfully complyed" with the request, this time for $5,000.

Finances were not made easy, even by this new loan. When James Wilson, Guardian, presented a bill for monies he had spent personally before the Committee had been formed, his account had to be disallowed. Still, so much more could the Committee of Distribution now do, and so much more was it asked to do, that on October 8 it was enlarged to eight members: Israel and Letchworth, Kerr, Mathew Carey (just returned to town), Swain, Haworth, Whitman, and Sharswood. Still later Savery and Benge were added, bringing the whole number to ten. This Committee of Distribution saved the poor from starvation. They distributed food, firewood, even clothes. They collected paupers and sent them to the Almshouse. Gratefully they learned that "friends in the country" were forwarding supplies and money to assist in the work.

Mayor Clarkson was particularly concerned with the financial crisis. When the New York City Committee for Quarantine and Relief wrote, asking what they could do, the Mayor answered frankly that, notwithstanding the calamitous situation, Philadelphia was abundantly supplied with necessaries and comforts. A few individuals had engaged to the Bank of North America; their "liberality upon the occasion is commensurate with our wants." The only worry he had, Clarkson added, was how the loans would be paid back. With this information, he left the citizens of New York "to exercise their benevolence in such manner as to themselves shall be most agreeable." Never was a cash gift solicited more delicately. The New Yorkers went right to work.

By the end of its fourth week, the Committee at City Hall was completely organized into subcommittees—the Bush Hill Managers, the Orphan House Committee, the Committee of

Distribution, the Superintendent of Burials and Removals (Samuel Benge), the Distributor of Supplies (Henry Deforest), and a few others. Of course, miscellaneous daily problems continued. One of the constant difficulties was finding enough room for burials. The graveyards looked like ploughed ground, Carey wrote, and Potter's Field was already more than full by September 28. A Quaker in town for a few days' visit looked at Potter's Field and exclaimed, "The half has not been told me!" Bush Hill's burying ground also could receive no more bodies after the end of September. The Committee considered carefully what should be done. Finally, they resolved on a step that was bold indeed.

William Penn's original plan for the city had included five squares of ground to be reserved perpetually as public parks for the citizens. "The North-West Public Square," between Eighteenth and Twentieth, Vine and Race streets, was in an almost uninhabited region of the city. It was also near Bush Hill. On September 28 the Committee sent two members to view the northwest public square, "and report the situation of it, and whether it would not be a more suitable spot for a burial ground than that now occupied for the purpose." They reported favorably, and the Committee instructed Joseph Ogden, sexton of Potter's Field, to inter the pauper dead in that square in the future.

To the Committee of Accounts (James Sharswood and John Connelly), expenses looked impossibly large. Both loans from the bank had been guaranteed by a popular subscription, but money to fill them came in slowly. From John Todd, Jr., a young Quaker lawyer, the first gift was received, $20, on September 16. That afternoon a cheque for $150 came from the merchants Thomas, Samuel, and Miers Fisher. Later that week came another five dollars, and the second week produced a $10 gift. The third week commenced with "four fine sheep for the use of the poor and sick," which Henry Deforest had to sell. Not until October 2 did contributions of any size begin to arrive. That day a letter from "sundry citizens" of Haddonfield, New Jersey, informed the Committee they had opened a subscription "for procuring supplies of provisions for the use of the sick and distressed" in the city: £80 had already been raised, forty-four fowls were being sent. Lownes published both the letter and the subscription, with the thanks of the Committee. Next day came a letter from New York City, which was also published. After that, contributions of money and gifts poured in regularly.

Carts laden with livestock, vegetables, supplies of all sorts came in over roads already thronging with refugees fleeing the city—from the Widow Grubb at Chester, eighteen bundles of shirts and shifts for the orphans; from Gloucester County in New Jersey, provisions regularly on the days before market days (and their subscription rose above £200), from individuals in the city, from committees and town meetings in Pottsgrove, Providence township, Salem, Woodbury, Mount Holly, Darby, and Evesham; from refugees like Commodore Barry who with others collected provisions and wrote to find how they could best send them in, from fugitives at Wilmington, Germantown, Norristown, and elsewhere, from Jonathan Williams at his farm "Mount Pleasant on the Schuylkill," from a host of towns, companies, and individuals. Each cash donation the accountants Sharswood and Connelly carefully entered in their books. Six men headed by Israel were named to parcel out the produce, clothing, livestock, and other goods of all kinds as they were needed. When the whole was totaled, the Committee was revealed to have spent over $36,000, some $3,200 more than they had received in cash; country donations had kept the deficit down to a reasonable figure.

IV

At the head of the Committee, Mayor Clarkson was responsible for the organization and efficiency of the whole body. The work of Israel, Lownes, Benge, Sharswood, Deforest, Letchworth, and all the others was given direction and effect by the

Mayor's continual firmness and quiet determination. The city's resistance was stiffened by his leadership and courage.

Soon the Committee had a census made of all closed houses, all infected, and all open, street by street. Later they compiled a list of all persons employed by them for public purposes, and a return of "the regular expences which the committee are at, in the prosecution of the business entrusted to their care; in order that a due oeconomy may be pursued in their expenditures." Still later they began to administer property left by deceased persons with no one legally authorized to take care of it. Conscious of public interest in their work as a governmental organization, they appointed Carey and Sharswood to select from their correspondence files such letters as ought to be published.

Of course, panic did not end in a moment. Throughout September continued the flights, the confusion, the demoralization, the pitiable discoveries of new nostrums and pious appeals to religious awakenings, the runaway apprentices, the escaped prisoners, all the other instances of dismay and disorganization. Closed houses and shops were invitations to burglary, so volunteers were called to add to the night watch—just in time, too, for the next night an attempt on the temporary post office was made, and barely frustrated. And people continually importuned or reviled the Negro carriers, until Mayor Clarkson publicly proclaimed that the insults, interruptions, and threats the blacks suffered would have to stop, or offenders would be punished. Public safety required that the Negroes be protected, and protected they would be, especially from those depraved persons who had no sentiments of humanity but such as concerned themselves.

Well-intentioned citizens continued to inform Editor Brown of all that needed doing. One urged burning tobacco in the streets. Another described a Russian recipe for fumigation concocted at Moscow. A third recommended earth-bathing. Still another declared he had cured himself by drinking two quarts

of molasses, which induced great bowel movements and discharges of wind.

Quicklime, gunpowder, whitewash, nitre, all had their champions. One writer urged that bedding be vinegared and buried
for three days in the earth. This would purify it.

Several citizens expressed concern over the condition of Philadelphia's privies. They stank, they were always near a well,
they were cleaned only once in ten or twelve years. A half-peck
of lime should be used in them right away, one writer said.
Another quoted "Moses the divine lawgiver" as to the proper
management of privies, and pointed out that persons in good
health used the same backhouse that received the foul wastes
from the sickroom. This was dangerous, the writer contended;
these "temples of Cloacina" were the very breeding grounds of
disease.

Yet gradually the work of the Committee made itself felt,
and such productions of panic began to recede into the background. The Committee, like the managers, were symbols of
the determination that arose within people to live with the
menace of the plague. And help was coming, now. The New
York committee had responded with splendid sympathy. Mayor
Richard Varick sent $5,000 to Clarkson as the contribution of
the Common Council of New York to Philadelphia relief. He
and his colleagues were, Varick wrote,

deeply impressed with the awful judgment of the Almighty on the
American Nation, in permitting a pestilential disease to lay waste
and disorganize that once populous, well regulated and flourishing
sister city, the seat of Empire, by destroying the lives of many valuable patriots and citizens and by driving many other of its numerous and very opulent and useful inhabitants into exile . . .

Acknowledging the "seasonable benevolence," Clarkson assured Mayor Varick that Philadelphians would profit by the
chastisement of the almighty disposer of events, "humbly kiss
the rod and improve the dispensation."

"Sangrado"

Never was the healing art so truly delightful to me. . . .—BENJAMIN RUSH, September 29

THE news of $5,000 from New York spread about the city like a tonic. It was, Editor Brown proclaimed, an act of noble disinterestedness, of sympathy and generosity. And as other donations poured in, the Committee wisely gave publicity to them all, even the smallest. Brown's columns soon were filled with letters from villages, townships, counties, congregations, and synods, all conveying gifts of some kind to the Mayor's care. The distraught citizens could take heart. They were not alone in misfortune. All America was sharing their burden.

That burden, meanwhile, was becoming easier to bear. Courageous leadership brought people out of panic to resolution, and beyond resolution to hope. With Girard and Helm at Bush Hill, with all the members of the Committee, with Mayor Clarkson and the humane Negro leaders, the citizens had plenty of examples of courage to emulate. And more than these, they had Dr. Rush.

Benjamin Rush had emerged from his ordeal of September 26 a man vindicated and restored, a man delivered from doubt. Once he accepted the fact of his sister's illness, and his mother's, he rose above his depression to still greater heights of service.

On September 29 he was tested by a new loss. Just as he was sitting down to write his wife, an old Negro coachman in the family of Samuel Powel called. His coach was outside, Dr. Griffitts was already in it. Would not Dr. Rush come at once across the Schuylkill? For Mr. Powel was very low. Rush went.

Mr. Powel was out of town in obedience to the Doctor's

195

directions. He had been ill; he had sent his family away; then Rush had ordered him to go also. Instead of joining Mrs. Powel, whom he might endanger, he had gone to a small house on a farm he owned west of town. There he convalesced. One day, unbeknownst to Rush, he had come back to the city to look after a servant who was ill. On his return to the farm he was seized again, very seriously. Mrs. Powel sent expresses twice a day to enquire for him. A young doctor of little experience attended constantly, but the Speaker lost ground so fast that the young doctor felt obliged to send for Rush and Griffitts.

The two friends, both thin and weakened by disease, their mouths dry and teeth discolored with mercury, were driven across the Upper Ferry Bridge and out to the cottage where Mr. Powel lay. Rush was dismayed to learn that the young practitioner had hesitated to bleed the patient a fourth time. With Griffitts, he spent all day and all night fighting for Mr. Powel's life, bleeding and purging. But he lost his battle. At six in the morning of September 29 the former mayor, speaker of the senate, and sterling patriot expired, in the bare little upper room of a tenant farmer. He died, Rush noticed, with a smile upon his face.

Brown spoke the general opinion, when he lamented Mr. Powel in the *Federal Gazette* as "a gentleman of benevolent disposition, and improved mind, a sound understanding, and an honest heart." To Rush it was but tragedy heaped upon tragedy. He returned home to find his sister much worse, perfectly composed, "prepared for her dissolution." He took to his coach, and visited thirty-one patients.

By October 1 Coxe was back at work, and Fisher expected to resume in a day or two. Rush seemed well; he gained strength every day. His mother, still complaining, apparently improved though she refused entirely to take the mercury purges or be bled. But his sister was declining hourly. On the first, she said to the Doctor, "A thousand and a thousand thanks to you my dear brother for all your kindness to me." At three that afternoon she breathed her last. Rush was deeply affected. "She had

borne a share in my labours," he wrote. "She had been my nurse
in sickness, and my casuist in my choice of duties. My whole
heart reposed itself in her friendship."

Half an hour after her death, Rush got in his carriage and
went his rounds of patients. Then that night, with his colored
Marcus, the mulatto boy Peter, and the Negro elder William
Gray, he followed his sister's body to the graveyard of Dr.
Sproat's church. "My heart has flown into the coffin with her,"
Rush declared to his wife.

The death of his sister on October 1 wrought a change in
Benjamin Rush. Though he tried to keep up his visits, and did
keep his house open to patients, his strength from this day forth
began to fail. All movement or motion became painful, his
appetite disappeared, night sweats returned, he had frightful
dreams. Time became meaningless to him. The days dragged
endlessly on, each one the same as every other. Once he saw a
man busily laying in wood for the approaching winter. "I should
as soon have thought of making provision for a dinner on the
first day of the year 1800," he wrote.

He was alarmingly frail. On the morning of October 4 he
suddenly fainted in the sickroom of a patient. He was carried to
his carriage, and had to stay at home the rest of the day. He
prescribed from his bed; Coxe and Fisher made his rounds for
him. Next day he was out again. His mother was improving, but
now little Peter, the mulatto boy, was infected.

On October 6 he had to refuse calls, but he went twice to Dr.
Griffitts, who was down a second time with fever. On the
seventh he visited Mrs. Meredith, but few others. Then on the
eighth he seemed restored and made many calls. Six other
doctors were ill; he was needed in the city. On the ninth he drove
himself harder than ever. That night he collapsed.

At one in the morning Rush was seized with all the symptoms
of the disorder. At two, after an hour's excruciating pain, he
called Marcus and Fisher. Fisher bled him, which removed the
pain, and gave him a dose and a half of the purge. "It puked me
several times," Rush wrote later; ". . . next morning it operated

downwards, and relieved me. . . ." For six days the Doctor was
prostrate, unable to see anyone but his servant, students, and
mother. These were the days of October 10-15. Fisher said he
had never seen so violent a case.

The gravity of his illness Rush concealed from his wife. Somehow he found strength to write each day; he mentioned that he
was confined, but said he was prescribing from his bed. Actually
he did not even sit up until the fifteenth, nor come downstairs
for several days after that. He did not go abroad until the
twenty-first. From the ninth till the twenty-first, the worst days
of all the fever, Dr. Rush was out of view.

Yet even in confinement he was, he wrote, still useful. Coxe
and Fisher brought him news every day; he directed their prescriptions. And as soon as he could sit up, he began again receiving patients in his house. Colonel Timothy Pickering, Postmaster-General, came to sit with him, to observe the stream of
patients and applicants thronging through the house, draining
the frail doctor's energies. He listened to Rush's account of his
methods, and of the conspiracy of other doctors against him.
Pickering believed it all. He sympathized.

Thus is a final clue to the riddle of Benjamin Rush supplied:
during the most critical days of the whole pestilence, he lay
alone in his room. Alone, that is, intellectually. He was assailed
with people, but they were universally his admirers. He was surrounded with assistants—his former students Woodhouse and
Mease, who now took cases for him, and Fisher and Coxe—but
they were his partisans. During all of October, Dr. Rush had no
conversation with any doctor his intellectual equal. Admirers
and partisans like Pickering served him not too well, for they fed
the flames of his quarrel, encouraged him in his delusion that
other doctors had confederated against him, brought him stories,
rumors, impressions that twisted the truth.

When he was sickest, Rush became most confident in his
method, most bitter against others. The confidence and bitterness alike etched themselves upon his soul; the impression never
disappeared. He saw the city's plight obliquely. The Committee

he pronounced a "forlorn hope." Bush Hill he declared a failure. All except mercury and jalap, and copious bloodletting, he condemned.

II

Now Rush was oppressively aware of the opposition against him, and against his method. All his confidence, all his faith, all the throngs of people who came to him, did not still the tempest in his heart.

Late in October he wrote in a burst of candor:

I am supposed to have created a great many friends, and a large fund of gratitude among my fellow citizens. This is far from being true. The relations and patients of the physicians whose practice I have opposed, have taken part with them in their resentments and I am now publicly accused at every corner of having murdered the greatest part of the citizens who have died of the present disorder. These slanders must increase, for ignorance and error when detected and exposed can *never forgive*.

He even considered moving to New York after the fever was over rather than remain in a city where he saw only strife and misery ahead.

Frequently as such depression seized him he despaired of ever winning over his colleagues. But not once during the whole plague did he ever imagine other remedies used by other doctors might be sound. Rush was impregnable in his fortress of error. Conscious of the purity of his life, conscious of meeting fantastic dangers without flinching, aware that many of his opponents had fled the city, Rush attributed their opposition to personal animus, to cowardice, or to envy. Resenting, with an intensity strengthened by illness, Rush began to make his own accusations of murder.

Those who opposed mercury and jalap were responsible for the continuing mortality of the disorder, he declared. In prejudice, fears, and falsehood they plotted against him. Scores were daily sacrificed to their bark and wine. "My method is too simple for them. They forget that a stone from the sling of David effected what the whole armoury of Saul could not do." Only those who adopted the great purge and copious bleedings were truly physicians. "The rest continue to murder by rule,—nor is this all, they have confederated against me in the most cruel manner, and are propagating calumnies against me in every part of the city."

Confederations, cabals, or calumnies were far from the minds of the other doctors. They were busy, as busy as Rush, with disasters of their own. But Rush could not endure their rejection of his revelation. In his tight little world of adoring patients, devoted students, admiring correspondents, he saw only his right and their wrong. Into his mind leapt fantastic suspicions, from his pen dripped a wormwood more bitter than his apothecaries ever knew. Ebenezer Hazard was not the only one who began to wonder about Rush. The merchant John Welsh deplored the difference among the doctors. He accorded "a monopoly of praise" to the Frenchman Nassy, who seemed to lose scarcely any of his patients, and as Rush's calomel and jalap failed to cure he observed the "great talk about it" dying away. When Rush first fell ill, Welsh believed he was not really sick, but only secluding himself to prescribe, mix preparations, and compose more newspaper essays. At the height of the plague he still pronounced Rush's opinions absurd, and toward the end he wrote that the mercurial purge was now held in the lowest esteem, particularly as it destroyed the coat of the stomach and bowels.

Joshua Dawson, Treasury clerk, heard around the city in October during Rush's second illness that the Doctor, "owing to the extreme fatigue of Body & Mind which he has lately undergone, is considerably deranged in his intellects for these two days past." The report persisted, and Dawson stopped Dr. Wistar on the street to ask exactly what ailed Rush. Wistar, he found, "seemed to wish to evade the enquiry."

Isolated, ill, sensitive, Rush paid for his convictions, his victories, his popularity with an epic torment in his soul. Self-confidence was not enough, or his great host of followers; he must have the unanimous support of the whole medical profession. This prize was never to be his.

As he recorded his torment, Rush grew sadder and angrier with his erstwhile friends and colleagues. Years before he had discovered how to treat lockjaw—large opiates, quarts and even gallons of wine and whiskey, quinine, baths cold and warm, oil of amber, salivation and blisters; that is, get the patient drunk enough and his jaw would drop, as drunken men's jaws always fell. But many physicians refused even to this day to accept his cure, and now with yellow fever they were proving just as obstinate. "If I outlive the present calamity, I know not when I shall be safe from their persecutions," he wrote Julia. "Never before did I witness such a mass of ignorance and wickedness as our profession has exhibited in the course of the present calamity. I almost wish to renounce the name of physician."

"Indeed," he added, "the principal mortality of the disease now is from the doctors."

The people would support him. Popular pressure had forced some of his most obdurate enemies to capitulate. "The people rule here in medicine as well as government," he observed proudly. And he remarked with even more pleasure that the fever was bringing people to God. An "evident sense of the divine goodness" pervaded those who had recovered. "Men now talk of God and of his providence who appeared scarcely to believe in either two months ago," he wrote, and begged Julia to continue to wrestle with God in her prayers. Meanwhile, he resolved not to falter. "I am in the situation of The French Republic surrounded and invaded by new as well as old enemies, without any other allies than a few of my old pupils, who are too little known to give credit to any innovation in medicine."

"But I am unmoved by the dull and wicked confederacy," he added. Even if they drove him from the city he would be happy, "wielding the plough with as much composure of mind as I now wield the lancet, or teaching a country school with as much pleasure as I have formerly taught medicine."

Ultimately, Rush's insistence on his method exerted a con-

siderable effect on his colleagues. Many accepted a moderate
form of his cure—bleeding and purging at the beginning of the
fever, bark, wine, and nourishing food as soon as the disorder
was checked. This compromise, Ebenezer Hazard said, was general by the end of October. But the victorious Rush was not
content. He was moved instead to distrust. Some doctors, he
wrote, offered "incense to the public mind" by one or two
bleedings and purgings, and then poured in their "poisonous
doses of bark and laudanum."

The "confederacy" against him grew so strong that Rush
feared "many, many persons" were killed by bark, wine, and
laudanum just to spite him. His enemies' rancor was boundless.
"They watch my patients with great solicitude and console themselves under my numerous cures, by declaring that my patients
had nothing but the common fall fever, and are all killed by
mercury and bleeding."

Murder "by large and ill-timed doses of bark and wine" he
could not prevent. It ended his professional friendships. "After
what has passed between me and the rest of them, we can never
consult, or even associate together."

III

In his charges of murder and madness, Rush passed through
every stage of animus, from pitying condescension to savage
abuse. The violence of his resentment increased, as the mortality
of the fever increased, and as illness and fatigue wore upon him.
On September 15 he had written that the contagion could be
eradicated if all would follow him, but instead doctors vilified
and slandered their only true guide. Then, as other physicians
began their public writings, he felt a great loneliness, and by
September 18 had fixed the blame on Kuhn—"learned and
sagacious" Kuhn, safe in Bethlehem. Kuhn left many patients
behind, whom Rush had to cure. Kuhn published his prescriptions, which Rush had to defeat. Yet Kuhn knew none of the
horrors of the plague. He was protected, while the nobler spirits
—Griffitts, Gibbons, Mease, Wistar, Leib, Penington, Carson—

were ill. Penington died; but Kuhn, in Bethlehem, could rise
every morning without facing the distresses of a doctor's waiting room, or viewing "the still more accumulated distress from
pain, fear, grief, poverty, solitude, famine, despair, and death,
which pervades nearly every house in the city."

Judge Lewis (himself safe in the country) gave Rush encouragement by an interpretation of Kuhn's motives. Kuhn, the
Judge wrote, had failed himself, and was jealous of Rush's success. He had either to admit himself wrong, or go on murdering
by rote. Unable to choose, he had fled the city and left his patients to shift for themselves. The country and town cashiered
him in their minds, Lewis declared, and were doing Rush full
justice.

Soon Rush realized that not as many doctors had adopted
mercury as he had believed. Nor were many more likely to do so.
Griffitts, Say, Leib, Porter, Mease, Physick, Annan, one or two
others—these were his friends. The rest, he thought, were
plotting together against him, directed by Kuhn.

"Even the nod of Dr. Kuhn in his lurking hole at Bethlehem,
commands more respect and credit from my brethren than nearly
1000 persons in different parts of the city who ascribe their lives
to the new remedies," he wrote.

William Currie—once his good friend—was "the weak instrument of their malice and prejudices." Currie with his pamphlet, his bark, his laudanum and cold baths, was one of the
conspiracy. Like Ross and young Barton and all the rest, Currie
had joined the "disciples of Dr. Kuhn."

"Disciples of Dr. Kuhn"—the phrase became Rush's curse. He
hurled it at one after another of his old friends as they persisted
in bark and wine. Dr. Johnson, in charge of the Dispensary, had
originally agreed with him about the French cure, but he would
not abandon Kuhn's fatally mild remedies, and he died of his
folly before September was over.

Worst blow of all was Wistar's "desertion." Wistar, on whom
Rush had depended, with whom he had consulted, for whose
life he had so diligently labored—Wistar, thought Rush, had

proved apostate. Actually the vague and lovable Wistar had taken no stand at all. He had only published an account of his recovery, paying tribute equally to Rush, Hodge, Parke, Kuhn, Carson, and his own students, Bache and Hart. All the doctors had benefited him, he said. But since he did not attribute his cure solely to mercury and bleeding, and since he confessed he had taken only half the doses Rush had ordered, his article confounded and amazed his friend.

At once Rush sent Wistar a protest. At a moment when the public mind was divided on the mercurial purges, he wrote, when "a thousand falsehoods were propagated against them," a word from Wistar would have turned the scale in their favor. It would have saved many lives. But instead Wistar had hesitated. "I considered your indecision," Rush wrote, ". . . a proof that you wished to stand fair with every body at the expense of—what, I shall not name."

Yet he felt, he added, "no disposition to resent being deserted . . . in the hour of danger and persecution by one whom I have loved like a brother—'Brutus as you know was Caesar's angel.' "

No one could have been more surprised than was the amiable Wistar at this letter. With no ideas of his own, he had merely hoped in his bumbling fashion to find everyone else's ideas in agreement. He replied plaintively, that he *had* acknowledged benefit from the mercurial purges, that he could not honestly have gone further. He recalled that Rush himself had not even known at the time whether mercury acted as an emetic or as a cathartic. He suggested that there was no magic about calomel— other medicines both emetic and cathartic might have been tried. He alluded delicately to the claims Rush had made that mercury had brought the disease as fully under control as the annual remittent. If so, he implied, why so many deaths? And he objected to receiving a letter full of "dashes and invectives."

But Rush could not forgive. Wistar's article had been, he declared, "calculated if not designed" to destroy confidence in his new remedies. Besides, it was inaccurate. He sent his own account of Wistar's case to Editor Brown, proving that mercury and bleeding alone had wrought the cure. It was an angry letter. Wistar, Rush had decided, headed the conspiracy against him.

"The most unkind attacks I have had," he asserted, "have come from Dr. Wistar and Dr. Currie, formerly my most cordial friends."

Later he heard that Wistar had treated his own brother Thomas (Dr. Hodge consulting) with mercurial purges and three bleedings in one day, but that pains had been taken to prevent the news of this reaching him. Again Rush pronounced Wistar a base trimmer, playing Brutus to his Caesar. To be Brutus twice in a few weeks (with Caesar still alive) was too much for Wistar. He complained that Rush was calling him an assassin. Rush rejoined that he was even worse than that. The puzzled Wistar wrote temperately to Brown's paper, describing his trial of bark, and the successful but too powerful operation of mercury in his case. "I do not write this by way of reply to Dr. Rush," he affirmed, "but merely to rectify what I believe to be a mistake in his statement."

It would, he added, be improper to take up a moment of Rush's time, that time so valuable to all the citizens, in argument. "I have ever studiously avoided newspaper controversy, and it would give me the greatest pain to be engaged in one, with a gentleman from whom I have derived a great part of my professional information, and whose friendship has been very beneficial to me."

But no soft answer could turn away Rush's wrath. After his second recovery he heard around the city that Dr. Currie had sent a letter to Dr. Hodge, filled with abuse of him, alleging he had introduced the mercurial purge only in order to make money by the sale of it. The letter was circulating among the confederated physicians, he understood. He asked Mease to procure a copy, so he could immediately publish it, to "shew that I had a more formidable monster than the disease, to contend with. . . ."

Of course, the letter never showed up. It had never existed. But the rumor was enough to turn Rush finally against Dr. Hodge. That sober gentleman, ever since the "discovery" of the yellow fever, had been laboring tirelessly all about the city, but Rush treated him with contempt. "This man has seen a great deal of the disorder," he wrote, "but he is no more the wiser for it than the black nurses who attend the sick. He is, if possible, duller than Dr. Kuhn."

When Hodge replaced him as Ebenezer Hazard's physician, Rush considered he had suffered one more blow than he could take. He addressed a brief letter to Dr. Hodge, and sent it to Brown for the columns of the *Federal Gazette:*

Dear Sir
  I regret that you & I differ so much in our Opinions & practice in the prevailing Epidemic, that it is impossible for us to consult together in any case whatever hereafter with Safety to a patient.
                           From Dr Sir your
                           friend &c
                           Benjn Rush

The appearance of this extraordinary communication, and the Doctor's daily letters describing the "confederacy" against him, gave Julia Rush in Princeton serious concern. She knew her husband's enthusiastic nature. She begged him not to indulge himself in controversies with other doctors. He wouldn't, Rush answered. He had started nothing. He had only "calmly contradicted their falsehoods." As for Hodge—he had given him "no other offence than declining to consult with him." This he would do to all other wine and bark doctors.

"A Jew and a Christian attempting to worship in the same temple, and by means of the same ceremonies, is not a more absurd sight than two physicians meeting to consult about a disease on the cause of which they differed as widely as light differs from darkness," Rush wrote his wife. He had not acted irresponsibly in declining consultation, he insisted. "I did not take this decisive step with my brethren till I made myself hoarse in trying to persuade them to adopt the new remedies, and until they had accused me in the news papers of murdering my patients by blood letting. The dye with them is cast."

"Well might David prefer the scourge of a pestilence, to that of the evil dispositions of his fellow men," the Doctor added.

IV

One searches Brown's *Federal Gazette* through all the plague
year in vain for those accusations of murder Rush insisted the
"confederacy" laid against him. Of course, Kuhn, Currie, and
the Frenchmen believed bleedings and the great purge dangerous, and said so. But actually many more favorable notices of
mercury and bleeding appeared than unfavorable. Letters from
patients bearing grateful witness to the success of Dr. Rush's
cure overwhelmed the few protests against it, and the small company of mercury doctors were as ready with the pen as with the
lancet. Rush magnified doubts into enmity; he also magnified
consent into virtue.

His greatest comfort, his highest reward, was the loyalty of
Samuel Powel Griffitts. Griffitts stood by him, "a Joab in the
present disease . . . fully in the new opinions and practice." Rush
conceived an affection for the pious little Quaker as intense as
his resentment of Wistar.

Griffitts was stricken ill in September, but recovered in time to
aid Rush at Speaker Powel's bedside. Then on October 6 he was
again confined. Rush bled him four times that day, but he continued very low. "O! what tugs are daily and hourly made upon
my poor threadbare heartstrings!" Rush wrote, after leaving
his friend. Yet three more bleedings improved Griffitts, and
finally in mid-October he was well enough to leave the city. He
sent Rush a parting note, which the Doctor at once despatched
to Brown's printers.

I am sorry to find that the use of the lancet is still so much dreaded
by too many of our physicians [Griffitts proclaimed] and while
lamenting the death of a valuable friend, I was this morning told
that he *was bled but once* during the disorder. If my poor frame,
reduced by previous sickness, great anxiety, and fatigue, and a very
low diet, could bear *seven* bleedings in *five* days, besides purging,
and no diet but toast and water, what shall we say to physicians
who bleed but once?

A younger man, Dr. James Woodhouse, only twenty-three
but already distinguished as a chemist, joined Rush's lists as

Griffitts fell ill. Woodhouse was saturnine, phlegmatic, somewhat bizarre; but he was Dr. Rush's protégé, and now he took
a great burden from his master's shoulders.

Dr. Peter Glentworth, a good mercury man, died on October
6, and by the eighth Rush had to note that Griffitts, Parke,
Currie, Physick, and Mease were all confined. Young James
Mease, after Hutchinson's death, had grown closer to Rush. He
was a convert to mercury. Twice he was seized with fever, bled
enormously by Rush, and twice recovered, though after losing
so much blood he was, Rush noted, a bit light in the head, and
"a mere skeleton." To Mease and Woodhouse Rush sent his
patients while he was ill, and on them relied for much of his
information. Mease, like Physick, Penington before his death,
and Annan, published testimonies of the effectiveness of the
great purge and bloodletting. And Dr. Porter announced in
Brown's columns that he saved thirty-seven patients in three
days by the new method. One case he had given up for lost,
Porter added, but a barber accidentally let sixteen ounces instead
of ten, and the patient walked away cured.

But Editor Brown also gave space to Dr. Thomas Ruston, a
once-skillful practitioner, former friend of Rush, now living in
the country. Ruston urged the mild remedy, warned against
bleeding and purging. Rush called this "reprobating his system."
He replied with a forthright article. Ruston came back with a
curious claim, namely, that he had discovered mercury and jalap
before Rush, that Rush had appropriated the credit to himself.
Now Ruston was twice foolish. He was writing from safety in
the country, and he was demanding credit for a method which
he impeached. "Do give that conceited fellow Ruston a severe
whipping," Judge Lewis wrote. Rush did, meanwhile confiding
to Julia that essays on the fever were coming "chiefly from
itinerant or fugitive doctors, or from a dull and profligate usurer
who has not seen a sick man these seven years."

Animus against Ruston was easily understood, but George
Logan of Stenton Rush had never despised. He had corre-
sponded with Logan regarding Parke's case and treatment of

the fever generally, and he knew that Logan was working devotedly in the city. But when Brown printed a column from the laird of Stenton, even though it endorsed bleeding and purging, Rush was scornful. He derided "Kuhn, Ruston, and Logan writing treatises on the yellow fever in their closets for the instruction of men who have gained a knowledge of it at hourly risk of their lives for four or five weeks." Others wrote to the *Federal Gazette* supporting Rush and condemning Ruston and Logan alike. "An Observer" declared Rush's method had nothing to recommend it but its success. Ruston said it would kill a horse, but it had cured a frail old lady in "Observer's" family. "A By-Stander" remarked that Dr. Rush visited more patients every day than Ruston or Logan had in fifteen years. And late in September appeared a terse paragraph:

The physicians of Philadelphia, engaged in attendance on those labouring under the pressure of disease beg leave through the channels of ye Gazette to present their compliments to Doctors Ruston and Logan, and request them to join them in active services, instead of insulting their understandings, and distressing the public mind by giving vain advice.

Logan, like Dr. Hodge, replied to no attacks, but (also like Hodge) kept right on working among the sick. Ruston prudently stopped writing by and by and remained in his well-merited obscurity.

Dr. John Linn, Rush's neighbor at 35 Walnut Street, died of the bark and wine. Old Dr. Redman, on the other hand, was open-minded, and took the mercury and bleedings as soon as he fell ill. So did Dr. Benjamin Say—"my much beloved and *tried* friend Dr. Say," Rush called him—and Dr. Robert Harris. But Dr. Samuel Duffield (the orphan-house doctor) insisted on being treated with Kuhn's regimen, even after his brother Benjamin had, Rush heard, adopted mercury and bleedings. Now Ben Duffield, busy at Bush Hill and converted to Devèze's methods, was actually following his own course. Rush was misinformed as to his conversion to mercury and bleeding, but the news he heard gave him keen satisfaction, for he was convinced that Duffield had "spent whole weeks in abusing those remedies and their advocates in every part of town."

Had he really known Duffield's practice, Rush would have received even greater hurt, for the French physicians and their notions were an abomination unto him. French treatments he thought even worse than bark and wine. They were the exact antithesis of his cure, in theory and application. French successes, even at Bush Hill (which he did not visit), he would never admit. He pointed out that "under the most favourable circumstances of accommodation and attendance" at the lazaretto, two-fifths of those admitted died. It was, he knew, because Devèze and Duffield failed to follow his way.

Rush would have had small patience, had he known of it, with Devèze's opposition to theories, his unwillingness to "force nature," his experimental attitude and varying treatment. For Rush, one disease demanded one cure. Many times in the city he was called in too late, he said, to save sick people who had been persuaded to employ French doctors. Jonathan Dickinson Sergeant ("I take as much pleasure in going to old enemies as to old friends," Rush wrote) was attended by two Frenchmen. So, Rush observed, he had "three chances against him to one in his favor—viz, a violent disease and two doctors."

The "new French Doctor," Robert, was prescribing for Miers Fisher. Citizen Robert was a high-spirited physician from Old France, who had lived a long time in, of all places, the Philippine Islands. When the French Revolution came, he decided to return home. A ship brought him around the world to Boston; there he heard of the fever in Philadelphia. He gave up a passage he had paid for to France in order to come to Philadelphia and help the suffering. He told everyone that bleeding and the mercurial purge were disastrous, probably fatal. He used a simple, gentle method, which he had long employed in the Philippines: barley water, tamarinds, gentle purges. He met with "uncommon success." But Rush, observing how he handled Mr. Fisher, pronounced Robert "equally a stranger to the disease, and to the principles of medicine." And at the end of October, when Bush

Hill had recovered many patients and with them its good name, when French remedies were in use even by many Americans, Rush still declared:

The French physicians are every where getting into disrepute. They have in conjunction with our bark, wine and cold bath Doctors, destroyed at least two thirds of all who have perished by the disorder. The principal remedies of the French physicians are hot baths, glysters, nitre, camphor and cream tartar. They seldom bleed and all of them reprobate the mercurial purges.

He added a curious story:

One of them (a Jew) does not even feel the pulse of his patients. Upon being offered a hand for that purpose by a Mr. Morrison, he said, "no—no. I never feel the pulse; that is the way the Philadelphia physicians catch the disorder." This man died on the 3rd. day.

v

The strange battle of the doctors, waged over the blood and vomit of the dying, disgusted those who were not won to Rush's course. "Benevolus" wrote complainingly to Brown's paper after the Rush-Ruston controversy:

For God's sake!—for the sake of those who daily wait for the publication of The Federal Gazette, with anxiety! and for your own sake! let your readers be no more pestered with disputes about a doctrine, which hath been a bone of contention for a couple of centuries, and at this moment as far from a decision, as when it commenced. Let the disputants have a little patience, perhaps the prevailing disorder will place them both in a situation to know more about the matter, than if they stay here for two centuries to come.

Others likewise objected, with pointed references to all the doctors' failures and to the mounting death toll. Again and again in the *Gazette* citizens appealed to the physicians to compose their differences. Dr. William Currie actually tried to do so. Like Wistar, he abhorred this controversy. Like everybody else, he recognized that it was discrediting the science of medicine itself. From his sickbed on October 2 he wrote a paragraph intended to be a compromise.

All the physicians in the city agreed with Dr. Rush, Currie announced, that bloodletting and copious purging were required "in every case where inflammatory symptoms are evident." The dispute had been, not over the proper mode of treatment, but over the name of the disease—this was what had caused all the fuss.

Now Currie meant this for laymen, and meant it to quiet their apprehensions that the doctors were all at sea. He knew that no professional man would fail to recognize how great an area was comprehended in that phrase, "the name of the disease." If you didn't name a disease correctly, you didn't have its nosology right, and therefore, of course, you couldn't treat it correctly. Nor could you understand what "inflammatory symptoms" signified when you saw them.

Dr. Rush, reading Currie's paragraph, interpreted it more simply. He called it Currie's recantation—declared he gave "full credit to bleeding and purging in the *yellow* fever," and added, "his and Kuhn's mistakes have cost our city many hundred lives."

But actually Currie had admitted nothing. Inflammatory symptoms did not appear in all cases. There were many fevers putrescent rather than inflammatory, there were many patients who exhibited both types of symptoms. To bleed and purge in putrescent cases where there was no excess stimulation of the arterial system would be fatal. Indeed, Currie had always maintained, every case was likely to be different, and had to be treated differently. He thought only a few of those ill in Philadelphia had the true yellow fever—perhaps forty or fifty out of the many thousands.

Rush, however, was inflexible on this point. He quoted every description of pestilence from Thucydides to Defoe, from Hippocrates to John Redman, to prove that one epidemic fever drove all other fevers out of a town. He even began to insist that the yellow fever drove out all other diseases of any type whatever.

Bleed, therefore, in all cases, he insisted. And purge. The variety of symptoms should not confuse the physician or becloud his understanding. The essential principle of medicine was the singleness of disease. "Intrepidity in the use of the lancet" was the only hope, he repeated. All fevers had one cause, and one treatment. No two epidemic diseases of unequal force could exist together. The yellow color was not an essential indication. The danger of internal rupture was increased because the hot summer had weakened people's blood vessels. When the sick showed no inflammatory symptoms, it was only because debility concealed them. Bleed and purge.

Bleed and purge, even when no symptoms of the yellow fever, or of any fever at all, appeared. Variety of symptoms were only "substitutes for the fever." Rush enumerated them: acute rheumatism, squint, stools white as in jaundice, sneezing and coughing as in influenza, tremors, twitching—these and all other symptoms only concealed the true disease, the single action of the miasmata. How wrong those physicians were "who found as many diseases in our city as the yellow fever had symptoms."

He ordered bleeding and purging for the son of Mordecai Lewis, but the disease proved stubborn in the boy's case. His vein would not close; it continued bleeding. The clyster would not stay long enough to operate. Every medicine strangled him. "We are left without hope," Mr. Lewis wrote. Suddenly the lad vomited up a great worm, eight or ten inches long, as thick as a quill. At once he felt better, and had a few hours of comparative comfort before he died.

VI

Now the battle of physicians was part of Philadelphia's great plague, part of community reaction to a death that stalked abroad in fetid mystery. Where all were confounded, some were bound to fight. Fighting was escape from defeat, scorn of mystery, a wistful reaching out for understanding. Had the doctors not contended, fever would have reigned supreme. By argument, they rose above dismay. A terror analyzed and described, a monstrous horror diagrammed, was fear reduced to reason.

Modern medicine is unanimous in condemning Rush's cure. Doctors today would approve the mild remedies used with success by Jean Devèze. But this is a conceit of superior knowledge. What vanities of today's science will not be repudiated in A.D. 2103? Historically, the right or wrong of the battle is an inconsequential matter. It is the fact of the battle that counts, rather than issues or results. The historian is a reporter, not a referee. He fashions his truth out of a whole syllabus of errors— errors that Devèze and Currie, Robert, Kuhn, and Hodge all made, as well as Rush. The historian's business is to understand, and to relate.

To understand the physicians is not difficult. Some, like Devèze, advanced into the unknown with tentative steps, observing every case and every symptom, proceeding from observed fact to hesitant generality. Had pride seized them, they might have described their method as true experimental science.

Others, like Currie, put to use every idea, every theory in the lexicon of medicine. They invented nothing, they conceived nothing, but with splendid learning applied the most and best resources of their profession. They represented all the dignity, all the prestige of conservative, traditional, informed medicine.

One, Dr. Rush, leapt beyond both fact and convention, that the vast fumes of tragedy might be destroyed by new strengths, new knowledges in the human mind. He alone passed the frontier, and many who saw him go took courage in their plight, glimpsed a new dimension of the spirit by which men live. Not all paths beyond the frontier lead to El Dorado. That Rush found himself in a swamp instead of a prairie detracts only a little from the inspiration his boldness gave, and still gives. And, in the long view, progress is made when explorers map the swamp. Those who come later have one less road to choose.

Benjamin Rush believed, very simply, that the human being was a whole and single personality, that one part of his body or soul could not be affected independently of all other parts. He abhorred the idea that there were many diseases. There was only one disease, though it might have many aspects. Just so, there was only one God, though he might be seen in many manifestations. Multiplicity of ills was as repugnant to truth in science as polytheism was to truth in religion.

The physician who considers every different affection of the systems in the body, or every affection of different parts of the same system, as distinct diseases [Rush wrote], when they arise from one cause, resembles the Indian or African savage, who considers water, dew, ice, frost, and snow, as distinct essences; while the physician who considers the morbid affections of every part of the body (however diversified they may be in their form or degrees) as derived from one cause, resembles the philosopher who considers dew, ice, frost and snow, as different modifications of water, and as derived simply from the absence of heat.

It was not unreasonable doctrine. Nor unchristian, nor unenlightened. It was only wrong.

But doctrine was a foolish matter to people who lay dying. They prized the human values. The afflicted saw many physicians working quietly, obscurely, faithfully, abjuring controversy and fame alike—little men, almost forgotten in the noise the great men made, forgotten by all but their patients. And they saw even the greatest, most contentious doctors, Rush, Currie, Hodge, all the noble train, go every day to the foul and stinking precincts of the sick. No one, however he mistrusted their skills, doubted the heroism and purity of "our Esculapians."

Yet there was one heroism that shone above all others. There was only one doctor who would enter a fetid chamber, scorn all protections, sit on the edge of a vomit-soiled bed, smile cheerfully to the frightened patient, say blandly, "You have nothing but a yellow fever." There was only one physician who could write in the midst of all his grisly duties, "Never was the healing art so truly delightful to me."

There was only one Benjamin Rush.

The Fugitives

Going out of town was, at least, going away from
the best medical help, and from a thousand con-
veniences, and perhaps necessaries, in sickness,
which only the city affords. . . .

—EBENEZER HAZARD

AMONG Quakers John Todd, Jr., was known as a promising
attorney, among members of his own family as a loyal son and
devoted husband. For so young a man, he had a lively social
conscience. His gift of $20—far more than a young lawyer
should have given—was the first contribution the Committee received, and in relief work among Friends he was tireless.

Four years earlier, John had married a lovely southern belle,
Dolly Payne, and installed her in a pleasant home at Fourth and
Walnut. One son was nearly two now, and in late August a sec-
ond son had come.

When the pestilence began, John moved Dolly, his son, the
new baby, and Mrs. Payne out to a farm home near Gray's
Ferry. He rode out to see them as often as he could, but in the
dreary waste of September days his duties in the city became ever
more confining. People needed lawyers: dying people to make
wills, survivors to settle estates, businessmen with contracts un-
fulfilled, debtors impoverished because there was no work. On
return day in court, John Todd was one of five lawyers present.
He looked about him, and remarked to Jacob R. Howell, a fellow
attorney, that they had better leave the infected region of the
Court House at once, for Samuel Benge's dreadful work of
burying the dead and conveying persons to Bush Hill was cen-
tered here in Chestnut Street. Howell was dead soon afterwards.

Among his unhappy clients John Todd labored ceaselessly, at constant risk and in dismal loneliness. He was much in love with his exciting wife; when his duties were over, he wrote Dolly, he would never leave her again.

Early in October his father, a schoolmaster in Chestnut Street, fell ill of the fever; so did his mother. John attended them both, but they died, and he followed their coffins to the graveyard.

Afterwards he met Friend Benjamin Smith of Burlington on the street, and in spite of the danger stopped to talk with him of the plague. He had passed on his way, when suddenly a thought occurred to him. He hurried back to Benjamin Smith. A scriptural passage had forcibly impressed itself upon his mind, said John Todd. It was this: "Be ye also ready."

He was ready. Sick in body and heart, he rode down to Gray's Ferry to his wife and children. At the doorstep, fainting, he gasped out to Dolly's mother, "I feel the fever in my veins, but I must see *her* once more." Dolly, still weak from her confinement, came down the stairs only in time to gather him in her arms. Thinking nothing of her danger, she laid him tenderly on a couch and watched over him. He died that evening.

For weeks afterward Dolly Todd lay close to death with fever, and the infection passed through her whole family. The new little baby died; but winter came on, and she and her older son recovered. They returned with her mother to the city, where Mrs. Payne began to take in gentlemen boarders. The handsome young widow of lawyer Todd was an appealing spectacle. Senator Aaron Burr certainly thought so, and he was accounted by all to be an excellent judge. It was Senator Burr who introduced Dolly Todd to Congressman James Madison of Virginia. That the distinguished statesman was twenty years her senior, even that he was a head shorter than she, did not long deter the lady of John Todd's heart. Eleven months after John's death Dolly married James Madison, and entered upon a career that would have amazed her simple, adoring Quaker lawyer. Dolly Madison's role in history began in the yellow fever of 1793.

John Griscom had his nineteenth birthday on September 27. It was mildly pleasant at nineteen to be a teacher in the famous Friend's School of Philadelphia, and no mean achievement for a Jersey farm boy, but the fever respected neither youth nor achievement. John Griscom fell ill. Painfully he made his way across the river and back home to Hancock's Bridge, below Salem, where he slowly recovered. Spared, Griscom went to head the Friends' School at Burlington, New Jersey, began to teach chemistry, later established the first high school in New York City, discovered the medical properties of cod-liver oil and how to treat goiter with iodine; he was in a great tradition of American chemistry.

Not so fortunate was Major Christian Piercy, a potter in Front Street at the corner of Artillery Lane. In September his son William, eighteen, was seized with the fever, and an apprentice, Isaac English, was likewise stricken. Alarmed for his wife and other children, Major Piercy crossed the river to Jersey to find a refuge for his household. On the stage from Camden to Salem he was suddenly seized with chills, fever, and nausea, to the consternation of other passengers. At a slight rise called Eldridge's Hill outside Woodstown he was forced to quit the stage. Isaac Eldridge would not take him in, but did grudgingly permit him to lie in an empty log cabin on his place. There, alone, Piercy died almost at once, on September 27, and was buried where he lay. In Philadelphia his son William died; the rest of his family sold all they owned and separated—not, however, before they erected a tombstone along the country road in Jersey to mark the Major's lonely grave. It recorded that Christian "Pircy" of the Northern Liberties, "aged 49 years 8 months and 27 days," lay buried there, and added for future riders of the stage the familiar warning,

> Stay Passenger see where I lie
> As you are now so once was I
> As I am now so You must be
> Prepare for Death and follow me.

Flight had begun as soon as panic; originally flight had been stimulated by the doctors' urgings. In the great northeast storm of Sunday, August 25, every road was jammed. So great was the terror, Mathew Carey wrote, that "for some weeks, carts, wagons, coachees, and chairs, were almost constantly transporting families and furniture to the country in every direction." Before the end of the fever, seventeen to twenty thousand people had fled the city, taking refuge wherever they could find a place. Half of the city's houses were closed in the height of the plague. If the fever was contagious, it was most certainly going to be carried into the country and to neighboring towns. Indeed, Thomas Rodney at Wilmington by September 15 was already hearing of many persons dying in the country who had caught the fever in the city. But if the disease was carried only by foul air, then country people had a chance of escape, for, Rodney was careful to learn, the air outside Philadelphia was not yet impregnated with the fetid miasmas of infection. "Yet," he added in a letter to his daughter, "the indignation of the Most High is very great and there is reason to apprehend that the distroying angel will lay waste the Country as well as the Cities before he depart—Let not your Mind Stray then from that which is right in his Sight . . ."

To those outside the city, where news had penetrated vaguely and in sporadic reports, the horrors of the plague were multiplied by a thousand speculations. As Judge Rush had found Reading full of contradictory rumors, so it was elsewhere. Every terrified fugitive added to the apprehension of the whole countryside within a week's journey of Philadelphia. It was no wonder that doctors in smaller villages, as fugitives trudged past their windows, sat down to write Benjamin Rush for firsthand news.

By mail, by mouth, and by that curious osmosis which spreads mass belief, the most exaggerated accounts of the city's plight were accepted, and frequently published in the papers. One New York gazette announced that the only business still carried on in the federal capital was gravedigging, or *"pit-digging,* where people are interred indiscriminately in three tiers of coffins." The *Maryland Journal* declared that 350 Philadelphians had

died in three days in mid-September; whole families were lost
in twelve hours, and the *Journal* quoted a Philadelphia correspondent as urging his Maryland friend to "use all possible
means to keep the fever out of Baltimore," especially to be careful about letting fugitives enter the Maryland city. A mechanic
wrote to a friend in Chestertown on September 5 that several
thousand had died of the yellow fever in the city, that "eight
thousand mechanics, besides other people," had left Philadelphia,
and every master in his branch of trade was gone.

Such rumors had their effect. Fear of contagion was universal,
and as fugitives streamed out of the city they were received with
alarm and apprehension wherever they tried to stop. Even paper
might contaminate. Postmasters in the country and in Jersey,
Maryland, and Virginia gingerly dipped Philadelphia letters
in vinegar with a pair of tongs before handling them, and
Brown's *Federal Gazette* was soaked and dried before many a
fire by distant subscribers.

The Santo Domingans in July had at least been given shelter
and food along the Delaware and Chesapeake bays, but fleeing
Philadelphians in September met frequently with brutal re-
ceptions, even persecutions. Some victims were, like Major
Piercy, forced to leave a stage and seek death on the roadside.
At Milford, Delaware, a wagon loaded with personal goods was
burned, the woman who owned it stripped, tarred and feathered,
and with a Negro servant run out of town. In Jersey a town
organized hourly volunteer guard duty to prevent any Philadelphian entering. At a southern seaport a ship from Philadelphia was refused wharfage, and obliged to stand out to sea
even without refilling its water casks; another vessel was stove
to pieces by the citizens.

At Trenton a man was "cruelly starved to death" because he
had been in an infected house in Philadelphia. A recently arrived
Irishman, walking west on the Lancaster Road, was enfeebled
by sickness and want. The people of the countryside would give
him neither comfort nor shelter, and taverns turned him out.

Finally, "oppressed by his calamity, and shocked by the brutality of his fellow men, he sunk down and died by a fence. . . ."

Ferrymen were able to enforce any rules and charge any prices. Some reaped an abundant harvest from the hapless fugitives. Carey heard endless stories of their heartlessness, and told them with relish. He learned also of a fugitive, ill beside a road, who lay calling for water until an old woman placed a jug near-by and told him to crawl to it. The man died, "and the body lay there in a state of putrefaction for some time, until the neighbors hired two black butchers to bury him, for twenty-four dollars. They dug a pit to windward—with a fork, hooked a rope about his neck—dragged him into it—and, at as great a distance as possible, cast earth into the pit to cover him." A fugitive lost his brother, but no cooper would make a coffin for him, so he was obliged to wrap him in a blanket and bury him with his own hands.

The Philadelphia stage was stopped two miles from Baltimore on September 17 by an armed guard. A near-by tavernkeeper refused to admit the twelve passengers, who huddled together at the roadside for eighteen hours. At Newark in Jersey a fugitive en route to Long Island was stricken and lay in the house of one Littel. The neighbors fenced in the house, blocked it off, and suspended services in a church just down the road. The man died, leaving a wife and small child. The widow would write a note every day stating what she needed and pin it on the fence; townspeople alternated in supplying her wants. At Bordentown a young Philadelphia girl deceived a sentinel by demanding, "Was *that there* confounded yellow fever got into the town?" The sentinel answered no, that she might enter Bordentown with as much safety as she would go into her own home, which of course she did. Another fugitive, located in a country village, lost his child with the fever, and went out to bury it. Returning, he found all his furniture on the road and the doors locked against him.

Stories of inhumanity of country folk to the fugitives were

told all about the city, and added to the horrors of the plague. "Ye unfeeling savages! Ye monsters in the shape of men!" wrote "A. B." in Brown's paper, after retelling a stickful of such anecdotes. "Remember that your judge will probably, one day say to you, 'I was a stranger and ye took me not in, depart from me ye workers of iniquity.' "

Numerous were the reports of contagion carried from city to town. However anti-Rush doctors might argue, no one could convince the country folk that the fever was not catchable from personal contact. "It is the plague, let them say what they will," wrote old Mary Norris of Chester, Dr. Logan's mother-in-law. And it had been brought in by those French sailors on the *Sans Culottes*— Mrs. Norris knew French sailors were the lowest kind of ruffians, who picked up all sorts of diseases from the Levantines.

Three members of the Hopper family in Woodbury, New Jersey, died as the result of aiding Philadelphia fugitives; so did a good woman in Chester County, and three people in one family in Trenton. A Negro servant of Mr. Morgan of Pensaucon Creek in Jersey fished an infected bed out of the Delaware, with the result that Mrs. Morgan and her daughter died. One of the Cadwalader family fled to his father's home in Abington, and communicated the disease. Yet Carey knew of many more fugitives who died without infecting anyone, even those who nursed them. He cited three at Woodbury, seven each at Darby and Germantown, eight at Haddonfield, and other instances at New York, Baltimore, Burlington, Lancaster, Newark, Bordentown, Lamberton, Princeton, Brunswick, and Woodbridge.

In all neighboring towns, panic as tense as Philadelphia's seized the people, and in every region communities followed Philadelphia's examples of prevention. As the stricken city had established quarantines against West India vessels, so all over the country in September quarantines began to appear against Philadelphians.

At Chestertown, Maryland, a public meeting on September 10 resolved that no stages should pass through the town, a committee of health was appointed, and a well-equipped isolation house set up to receive fugitives. Chestertown's action regarding the stage was enough to cause the Eastern Shore line to suspend operation altogether in a few days. The Western Shore coach to Baltimore soon found at Havre de Grace constables refusing to permit anyone to cross the Susquehanna who could not show a certificate proving that he had *not* come from Philadelphia, or any other infected place; and on September 13 a public meeting in Baltimore prohibited citizens from receiving in their houses any fugitives unless they had previously been examined by the health officer. Next day the Maryland militia occupied a post on the Philadelphia Road two miles above Baltimore, to keep out all infected, or any who had been in Philadelphia within seven days. By the nineteenth the Western Shore stage had ceased to run.

Soon Baltimore added other restrictions, prohibiting the importation from Philadelphia of goods capable of carrying infection (and what were not?) and banning all the baggage of travelers. The Governor of Maryland proclaimed a quarantine of forty days against all Philadelphia vessels, and set up border guards against immigrants by roads. As far out west as Hagerstown, ordinances were passed interdicting all traffic in goods and people with Philadelphia.

In Virginia on September 17 the Governor ordered a twenty-day quarantine of vessels, Alexandria stationed a lookout boat a mile off the town to stop and examine ships, and Winchester placed guards on all roads to arrest every person, package, or conveyance coming from Philadelphia.

In another direction, at Trenton and Lamberton, citizens prohibited any Philadelphian crossing the river by ferry, and banned all traffic by water with the capital city from the Jersey towns, including Lamberton, Trenton, and Bordentown. Any persons from Philadelphia or Kensington already on the Jersey shore were ordered to leave.

Mayor Richard Varick of New York City on September 11 wrote all physicians in his town requiring the names of patients recently come from Philadelphia, and ordering them removed from the city if they suffered an infectious disease. A hospital had been set up; but Mayor Varick observed that no power in the state could lawfully interrupt commerce with Philadelphia. Governor Clinton next day established a quarantine of the port, stopping all vessels by sea from Philadelphia at Bedloe's Island, but he also found no lawful power to interdict passage across the Hudson River. A meeting of citizens in the city showed no such legalistic scrupulousness. They hired two physicians to assist the port examiner, directed that overland (Jersey) traffic be checked as much as possible, and wrote the proprietors of the southern stages that the inhabitants earnestly desired their boats and passengers should not pass during the prevalence of the fever in Philadelphia. Later the same week (September 17), the city council resolved to stop all intercourse with Philadelphia entirely, and posted strong guards at every landing to send back anyone from the stricken capital.

General Henry Knox, the Secretary of War, had been placed in charge of the government by Washington when he left Philadelphia on September 10, but after a few more days of the plague, Knox deemed it prudent to depart. He reached Elizabethtown on September 19, after the New York quarantine had been established, and was forced to remain more than four weeks in the Jersey town. So many less conspicuous fugitives, however, stole across to Manhattan in spite of the guards, that on September 23 a night watch of ten citizens in each ward was posted, and a strong published address urged all inhabitants not to take strangers into their homes. Regulations were printed requiring goods from Philadelphia to be unpacked and aired forty-eight hours before coming into the city, and bedding washed and "well smoked with the fumes of brimstone."

Still, fugitives somehow entered the town, and on October 11 the council threatened to publish "as enemies to the welfare of the city, and the lives of its inhabitants" all who attempted to import Philadelphia goods. Even after the fever ended, attempts to bring beds, bedding, feathers in bags, or secondhand clothing to New York were prohibited.

Fat and jolly General Knox amused himself during his tedious quarantine at Elizabethtown by describing New York's panic to President Washington. The militia was out all over North Jersey, he wrote, and from Manhattan Island reason had entirely fled. Philadelphia fugitives were frightened to death by being interned on Governor's Island without proper accommodation. One boat from Jersey landed passengers in New York, but a mob collected and insisted that the newcomers were infected. They forced the passengers back on board, and among them drove one of their own number, a New Yorker named Mercier. Mercier pled in vain that he had not been away from the city for a long time. The mob, nevertheless, refused to let him come ashore, and Mercier had to spend the night on board with people he was sure were feverish.

Knox told also of a New York tailor who had the common fall fever. He took Rush's medicine so often that he grew really ill, and though a Newark physician said he had only the autumnal disease, people ordered his coffin in his presence. And, "to mark the monstrous absurdity which prevails the people came into the sick man's room in shoals to see *the curious fever,* and he has been so worried that his life is in great danger."

The Secretary of War had pressing business at home in Boston, and was anxious to continue his journey. After all, he only wanted to pass through New York, not to visit there. He tried to get a boat to Newport, but none would take him. Newport was full of rumors; popular report was already saying that forty died every day in New York City of the Philadelphia fever. Impatiently the General finished his quarantine. He was, he remarked ruefully, "too bulky *to be smuggled* through the Country."

In still more distant ports, fear of infection caused similar restrictive measures. In Massachusetts the legislature passed a health law authorizing inspection and purification of persons, baggage, merchandise, or effects, and the selectmen of Boston proclaimed a twenty-one day quarantine of vessels and immigrants from Philadelphia. During the three weeks of their quarantine fugitives' baggage or merchandise should be "opened, washed with vinegar and fumigated with repeated explosions of gunpowder."

Newburyport made similar regulations, and the Governor of Rhode Island issued a proclamation enjoining vigilance and strict enforcement of existing laws.

In the south, North Carolina established a state-wide quarantine of vessels. Newbern laid fines of £5 for white men, plus fifty lashes for slaves violating the regulation. South Carolina likewise instituted quarantine, while the city of Charleston forbade any vessel from the Delaware River to cross the harbor bar. Georgia obliged all Philadelphia vessels coming up Savannah River to lie in Tybee Creek until inspected, and Augusta passed preventive measures. It was inhuman of other cities to take advantage of Philadelphia's distress, Ebenezer Hazard wrote Jedidiah Morse—inhuman to proclaim how healthy they were, and refuse asylum to the fugitives.

Commercial losses were immense, both to Philadelphia shippers and to merchant houses in other ports. From Philadelphia wharves in the previous twelve months no less than seven million dollars' worth of goods had been exported—a quarter of all America's outward shipping, twice as much as went each year from any one state. To Philadelphia had come in twelve months 1,414 vessels, 477 of which were ships and brigs. But now the port, like the city itself, was empty, and goods rotted where they lay in the countinghouses up and down Front Street. Commercial losses were not offset by days of fasting, humiliation, and prayer proclaimed in nearly every American town, or by the extensive gifts of money and provisions collected everywhere for Philadelphia.

Nearer the plague center less stringency was observed, partly because fugitives from Philadelphia meant a boom in local trade, partly because towns on high ground were confident of the salubrious quality of their atmosphere. Even Chester, low as it was, remained fairly healthy; few died, and those all sailors or fugitives from the city infected before they came. Everyone had suitable nursing and attendance, and apparently the infection did not spread. There were alarms, however. Mary Norris observed that a waterman from down river died, some thought, of the yellow fever, though Dr. Preston said he died of too much rum; the cautious inhabitants buried him immediately. Chester offered asylum, though a somewhat uneasy one. When the Hoskin sisters, already ill, came down river, the shallopman who brought them was discharged by his employer, who had given orders to carry no passengers from Philadelphia. Even the owner refused to go on board the shallop after it had discharged its burden.

The town of Reading banned trade, admitted fugitives only after examination, and discontinued the stage on September 24. Bethlehem and Nazareth resolved upon a twelve-day quarantine, but did not enforce it. At Easton fugitives were merely asked to isolate themselves for a week from the local inhabitants, crossing the Lehigh River to do quarantine. Yet in these towns there were serious cases. The judges of the Supreme Court recorded numerous observations of fever as they made their September circuit. Chief Justice McKean, who had been gravely ill, recovered in time to go to Lancaster for term, though he lived entirely on a liquid diet of wine and whey.

Judge Bradford saw fever in every little village, and when he reached Easton observed the death of a ferryman of that town. The frightened citizens threw the poor chap into a grave within fifteen minutes, causing Bradford to wonder if he was really dead when the earth fell upon him. At Easton, Bethlehem, Reading, and Lancaster, Bradford heard accounts that grew ever more sensational. Letters at such a time were like cool water to a thirsty soul, he wrote; yet he confessed he behaved as a coward every time a letter came, fearing the news it would bring. In some ways it was almost as frightful to be away from the city as to be in it.

A few towns proceeded with extraordinary generosity. Woodbury, New Jersey, allowed free entrance; Elizabethtown and the
near-by village of Springfield actually offered their hospitality
as asylum, though they did not, as Phineas Bond suggested to
Elias Boudinot (Elizabethtown's most distinguished citizen),
offer premiums and bounties to their doctors and nurses who
would volunteer to go to the capital city. Elkton in Maryland
followed the example of Chestertown in preparing a hospital.
Most helpful of all was Wilmington. In spite of its riverbank
location, the Delaware town on its noble hill was (for once)
free of disease. Philadelphians by the hundreds flocked there,
houses were jammed, rents rose to the sky; Christina Creek
was black with vessels of all kinds, every inch of wharf space
was filled with ships discharging passengers, baggage, and
crews. A young Englishman, William Cobbett, was living in
Wilmington at the moment, teaching English to the French
refugees. "We hear that all Philadelphia is dying," he wrote to
a friend, and added that if the sickness continued Wilmington
would be a seaport indeed, "for we have here at present seventeen or eighteen merchant vessels, which come here instead of
going to Philadelphia." At first, Delawareans were appalled at
the spectacle. Every inn except Brinton's closed, quarantines
were established and guards posted. Then Dr. Way, Major
Bush, and other citizens began publicly to receive fugitives; soon
the whole town was welcoming them, and a hospital was provided—though it was little used, for Wilmington people preferred to nurse the stricken in their own homes.

As stages suspended and vessels were quarantined, fugitives
found it ever more difficult to leave the city. Dr. Rittenhouse
stayed at home until his son-in-law, Jonathan Dickinson Sergeant, died. Then he took his family in his own coach out to his
Norriton farm. Those who depended on public conveyances,
however, were often stranded.

A more serious effect of the quarantine was the end both of
commerce and news. The result of the first was the collapse of
Philadelphia's economy. The absence of money became a serious

handicap to the city. Prices rose out of reach, and lack of trade prevented new supplies of cash from entering the market. One bleeding cost seven shillings six pence, and medicines were so dear that few could afford them. Dr. Rush advised a rich man to send to the apothecary for a mercurial pill; the patient confessed he had no money, and begged the Doctor to give him one from his shop. Rush himself was frequently embarrassed for lack of funds. His brother-in-law sent him $100, which was, as he put it, "very acceptable." The rent of a carriage alone cost him $6 a day, laundry seven shillings sixpence per dozen, apples two and six the half-peck, and though he was "so ragged, that I am hardly fit to be seen in my own house," he could find "scarcely a Taylor or Shoemaker who carried on business in town, their apprentices and journeymen being dead, or turned grave diggers, or having left the city." Debby Logan at Stenton found that she had worn out all her shoes, but she dared not send in to the city to procure new ones, and doubted anyway if they were to be had. The want of news was even more serious in its moral effect, both on those who remained and on the fugitives who could hear nothing accurate of their friends and families in the city.

Thomas Boylston Adams, son of Vice-President John Adams, was studying law with Jared Ingersoll, Pennsylvania's attorney-General. For some while he stayed in the city; then he went to Woodbury, New Jersey, where he and his friend Mr. Freeman were the first arrivals. He chose Woodbury because every village on the Pennsylvania side of the Delaware was crowded with deserters, but Woodbury, near as it was, seemed fairly quiet. Many followed Adams and Freeman, each bringing news of the city. Thomas sent his father word of Jonathan Sergeant's death, and complained of his lack of winter clothes. At Woodbury he stayed fully ten weeks, isolated from the world in the Jersey meadows and miasmatic swamps. He missed the newspapers:

I don't know that I ever experienced the value of Public prints, by the want of them before now. Hereafter I shall always be opposed to the tax upon Newspapers. . . . The minds of the people have been so much agitated by the disease in Philad'a that no one gives the least attention to politics or government.

He heard that Pennsylvania had held an election, in spite of the fever, and that Mifflin had won.

Dr. Rush deemed the isolation and quarantine of each village prudent and wholesome. When he learned that Trenton had suspended intercourse with Philadelphia he advised his wife she need not seek refuge further away than there or Princeton.

Nearer the city, the presence of fugitives had created strange scenes of crowding, resentment, and charity in every town and village. All the houses and barns around Gray's Ferry, or down in "the Neck" below the city, over the Schuylkill, up the Delaware, or along the Ridge Road, had their quota of "deserters." Phineas Bond, the British consul, retired to Moore Hall, his seat in Chester County; Bishop White sent his family to his farm below Media ; in the Northern Liberties, at Falls of Schuylkill, in Jersey, up the Delaware, and in Germantown the gentry sought their relatives and friends.

Germantown, strangely uninfected, was the closest, and soon became the most crowded, resort of the fugitives. When Judge Bradford returned from circuit he stopped at Falls of Schuylkill to dine with the Governor. Mifflin was completely recovered, he found; he "takes wine as well as ever." Edmund Randolph was living east of Germantown, while to the west was Oliver Wolcott at Provost Smith's enormous home above the Falls. Every house was filled with people, every store building occupied with Philadelphia firms. Germantown was collecting relief funds at a great rate, even though the inhabitants made every effort to keep the infected out. Little help was given the sick, nor were the dead welcome in the graveyards. One victim had to be buried in the orchard back of the house in which he died. When Jacob Hiltzheimer rode out from town on the day deaths first passed one hundred, he found the fugitives anxious to learn the news of the city, but fearful of coming close to him when they found he had come from downtown. For Elizabeth Drinker, Germantown seemed to hold fully half of Philadelphia, and to wear a carnival aspect. A great crowd gathered to watch the immersion ceremonies of the Dunkers' church in the Wissahickon, and the whole town turned out one night when Livezley's mill caught fire and burnt to the ground.

The Northern Liberties were likewise healthy, and to the great homes above the city all who had some entrée fled. Stenton was filled with Logans, Norrises, and other connections of Dr. Logan and his lively Debby, and when Judge Bradford reached home at Rose Hill he found the "family" safe and healthy, though almost entirely uninformed concerning affairs in the city.

At Frankford village, on the other hand, business was booming, and Philadelphia's misfortunes were closely watched, for many of the import-export merchants moved their stores to Frankford and carried on their trade from there. Miller & Abercrombie, Samuel Pleasants & Son, Robert Smith ("at my house back of the Jolly Post tavern"), and numerous others found the up-river town both healthy and convenient. Some merchants, like the apothecaries Betton & Harrison, opened stores in the Northern Liberties and Germantown, while many advertised goods for sale at the wharves in Wilmington.

Those in the city, meanwhile, were quick to note the flight of every prominent person. Dr. Ashbel Green, minister of the Second Presbyterian Church, had gone with his family to Princeton in August to see a sick child, and was then called further away to a dying brother-in-law. By that time Philadelphians were "flying in all directions," and Green deemed it prudent (after consulting Dr. Rush) not to return. Frequently about the city Rush heard Dr. Green censured for deserting his post, but always did him "ample justice" by openly declaring he had advised the reverend gentleman to stay away. Dr. John Ewing, distinguished provost of the University, rector of the First Presbyterian Church, and secretary of the American Philosophical Society, "consulted his safety by removing early," as Ebenezer Hazard pointedly remarked; so did Dr. Samuel Magaw of St. Paul's Episcopal Church; and neither received any quarter from their deserted parishioners. When Rush heard that Magaw was in the country he hoped it was true, for Magaw was a good man, in the Doctor's opinion, "and I think would not have left his flock had his health permitted him to remain with them."

Yet in spite of doctors' advice and the obvious reasonableness of flight, most of those who stayed had harsh words for those who fled. They were called deserters, malingerers, profiteers, renegades, and cowards. The absent doctors particularly were despised, and by others than Rush. Ebenezer Hazard wrote bitterly of Shippen and Kuhn: "their fears have made them *fugitives* at present," he told Jeremy Belknap. "May you never want *their* aid!"

Actually, Mathew Carey pointed out, the fugitives suffered in many ways just as much as the hardy spirits who remained. Half of Philadelphia was in the country and not half of Philadelphia were blackguards. Fugitives were prey to all manner of hardships and privations; they suffered the tortures of uncertainties and lack of news; furthermore, they performed a service by leaving. As "the nature of our government did not allow the arbitrary measures to be pursued, which, in despotic countries, would probably have extinguished the disorder at an early period," Carey observed, those who could avoid the disease by flight saved the city and the doctors much labor by their departure. Empty houses stopped the progress of disease on every street; absent mouths prevented famine.

"Let those then who have remained, regard their long-absent friends, as if preserved from death by their flight. . . ." Carey concluded; "Let those who have been absent, acknowledge the exertions of those who maintained their ground."

Height of the Plague

OCTOBER

The same melancholy scene of devastation continues! Whoever are the survivors will be shocked at the altered appearance of the city.
—DEBORAH NORRIS LOGAN

EVERY day was like Sunday, Ebenezer Hazard wrote, the streets deserted, houses shut. When friends met their conversation was always: What deaths today? Burials were quick, businesslike affairs, with no clergyman, no ceremony—"the putrid Corpse is committed to its kindred Earth, & covered up as expeditiously as possible."

Fully seven members of Hazard's family were down at one time: he, his wife, daughter, a serving girl and a serving boy, a German indentured girl whom Hazard had lately purchased, and an ancient female connection. Dr. Hodge made daily visits, and under his ministrations all but the ancient female connection recovered. Occasionally, Hodge would sit and talk, resting from his endless rounds, speculating on the disease. It had changed its nature since the beginning no less than four times, he reported. Now its malignancy was greater than it had ever been, it was more fearsome, relentless, almost irresistible.

It was the dismal monotony of the plague that everyone found so hard to bear—yesterday's desperate losses, today's doomed cases, tomorrow's inescapable tragedies. The mind could conceive no hope or encouragement. Some observations promised greater disasters to come. One young doctor pointed out that a calm day, or a westerly wind, brought an increase of deaths, that

233

sunlight was harmful, that electric fluids in the air (such as the aurora borealis observed one night) were invariably fatal. Whenever the barometer fell people died, and worst of all, as October began, was his proof that the time of the new moon was the most dangerous.

In September, over fourteen hundred deaths had been recorded. For two weeks burials had amounted to more than seventy a day. Then the new moon came. At first, October showed the same average of seventy; but on Monday the seventh, eighty-two were buried, on Tuesday the eighth, ninety, on Wednesday the total passed one hundred, on Friday, October 11, it reached one hundred and nineteen. The worst of the plague had arrived.

II

The dusty stillness of the streets was frightening by day, for along those empty ways the poisoned miasmata stole about, creeping invisible through doors and even walls, seeking the bowels of every living thing. Here and there lay the rotting bodies of dead cats, destroyed, people supposed, by the same pervading morbidity in the atmosphere that destroyed all life.

But nights were far worse, the melancholy silence of the nights in which rode the pale sliver of the new October moon. Through the awful loneliness of night the Reverend J. Henry C. Helmuth of the German Congregation trudged "with a trembling heart," going from one victim to another, raising fearful din in the silent city as he lifted a door knocker, radiating saintly calm as he entered a sickroom, facilitating many a passage into eternity. Down streets empty as a wasted desert, past boarded shops and closed houses, for two and three dark squares he would meet no human being, hear no sound but the doleful creaking of the dead cart as it went its ceaseless rounds.

In the morning, doors slammed and windows closed as a coffin went by, accompanied only by the "inviter" and a sexton. In one block of Appletree Alley Parson Helmuth counted nearly forty dead. But tragedy among the living was more affecting even than death. Cries, shrieks, and lamentations greeted him as he entered a house. People found release in Helmuth's gentle presence. They wept, they fainted; and between times they bespoke of him coffins and graves for their sick. Such haste to be rid of suffering human beings, such unseemly beforehandedness in arrangements of death, shocked Dr. Helmuth. He was learning much about the human mind. Madness, he observed, was common, among the well as much as among the stricken.

Helmuth had a formidable question to ponder as he made his weary way about the city. Fully twice as many of his Lutherans were dying as Quakers or Methodists or Catholics or members of any other church. The saddened Rector could not but wonder why. He reflected that his people were poor, and suffered most thereby; few could leave town, hence they were the more exposed. But the real reason, he concluded, was that his Lutheran cemetery was the easiest of all to be buried in. The congregation's licenser of graves had fled early in the plague, and the inviter of the dead was continually busy at funerals. The congregation had instructed him to permit any burial gratis, without asking the faith of the deceased. While he was busy he left a little boy of nine at the cemetery gate to give anyone who applied tickets for Martin Brown, the gravedigger. This became known. And it was also told about the city that the Lutheran inviter and driver would put a body into a coffin with their own hands. As a result, hundreds who had never been inside the chapel came to the German cemetery with their dead. Later Dr. Helmuth wondered just how many of the 641 new graves opened in his tiny burial plot between August and November contained the mortal remains of people who had some reasonable right to be there.

Still, for all his rationalizing, Helmuth knew his losses had been enormous. In six days—October 6 to 12—130 of his flock perished. God's judgment upon him was hard. Now his colleague, the Reverend John Frederic Schmidt, had the fever; and Martin Brown, the gravedigger, and his mother had died.

To so many dangers was the conscientious Dr. Helmuth

exposed that he emerged, Mathew Carey declared, a living
miracle of preservation. The same could be said of the Rev. John
Dickins of the Methodist Church, of Thomas Ustick of the
Baptist Meeting, of old Mr. Annan of the Scots Presbyterian
Church (Dr. Annan's father) and Bishop White, who "stood
to his post."

But others who likewise did the works of mercy and grace,
visiting the sick, comforting the afflicted, feeding the hungry,
confessing the dying, were not spared. Small wonder, as one
minister after another fell ill and even died in devotion to his
pastoral care, that the reverend fugitives Ewing, Green, and
Magaw were reviled on the streets. Joseph Pilmore of St. Paul's
Church had to take Magaw's burdens as well as his own. He
was found "everywhere, where there is sickness and distress,"
until he was stricken, and for days hovered in a perilous condition, cared for by Dr. Annan.

Dr. Robert Blackwell, rector of St. Peters, stayed until he
collapsed; then his wife conveyed him to Gloucester in Jersey.
Rush sent young John Coxe every day to bleed and purge him,
and had Woodhouse go along too when he could. It was a near
thing. Blackwell could not be nursed half so well in Gloucester
as he could have been in his own house in town; and Mrs.
Blackwell was continually advised against bleedings by a friend
who had been a patient of Dr. Kuhn. But she was firm in her
loyalty to Rush, and Coxe was avid with his lancet; the good
man recovered. Rush, having received many notes and bulletins
from Mrs. Blackwell, finally was able to write congratulating
her on the Doctor's recovery under the care of two young physicians, a signal triumph of "youthful reason and experience, over
grey headed ignorance and error."

The absent Presbyterian ministers were so much criticized
that the Reverend John Blair Smith sent a long letter to the
Federal Gazette resenting imputations against him and his colleagues; and "A. B." observed in defense that, since they were
Calvinists, the Presbyterians must have survived or perished
according to God's scheme anyway, whether they stayed or fled.

The venerable Dr. James Sproat of the Second Presbyterian Church was hard pressed because of the flight of Green, Smith, and Ewing. The fever was vicious in the toll it took of Dr. Sproat as he labored in the city. His younger daughter died on September 23, and the feeble old man tottered along after her coffin, weeping as he committed her to the grave. His son succumbed a few days later, and by the middle of October the good minister himself had been struck down. Dr. Sproat "finished his course," Rush wrote, the morning of the eighteenth, and that afternoon Philadelphians beheld the almost forgotten spectacle of a public funeral: more than a hundred people, chiefly women, followed the beloved preacher's coffin (borne by eight Negroes of the African Church), and at the grave the Reverend Joseph Turner, an Episcopal rector, exhorted them in a sermon. Mr. Turner subsequently was desperately ill.

In the Catholic cemetery by the middle of September more than two hundred new graves had been opened. All the Catholic priests in the city were infected. Father Francis A. Fleming, vicar of the Northern District under Bishop Carroll of Baltimore, was an Irishman, a Dominican, formerly rector of the Irish College at Lisbon, who had come to Philadelphia late in 1789. Everyone liked him. He was friendly, kind, exceedingly learned. Catholics said he was bound to be a bishop. In a spirited public controversy with the Reverend Robert Annan in 1792 Fleming had written an exposition of the doctrine of papal indulgences, thus becoming one of the first American pamphleteers in a Catholic cause.

On September 10 Fleming made his will. Then by a fleeing parishioner he sent a letter to Bishop Carroll, informing him that he, Father Keating, and the "worthy bishop-elect" had so far escaped the pestilence. The worthy bishop-elect was the German Father Laurence Graessl, a forty-year-old Bavarian, formerly a Jesuit, who had come to what he called "midnightly America" six years before and, as he put it, had wandered a great deal in the American forests to gather the scattered sheep. His knowledge of languages served him well in the capital city.

He heard confessions, many of them, he said, in German, English, French, "Welsch," Dutch and Spanish. It was inspiring to be a pioneer priest in the new world. But suddenly in the summer of '93 a new responsibility was thrust upon him. "There is but one bishop in this extensive country," he explained to his parents back in Bavaria.

Should he die, another of the clergy would have to travel to Europe to receive the episcopal consecration. Therefore, the Pope gave permission to select a coadjutor-bishop who should succeed our worthy bishop. The election took place in the beginning of May and, dearest parents, the choice fell on your poor Laurence.

To be first coadjutor of America's first Catholic bishop—this was no small distinction. Almost immediately, however, Father Graessl contracted malaria, and was convinced his life was about to end. The news of his election as bishop coadjutor, coming as he felt himself dying, brought him disquiet and dismay. "Pray for me that God my strengthen me in my last fight," he begged his parents. "Pray for me."

Yet by September Bishop Graessl was recovered and back at his duties, preparing to assume the burdens of the bishopric. Not nearly so well known in the city as Fleming, he was none the less effective, and both priests, together with Father Keating, moved about town day and night continuously in the service of the sick of all religions. One after another they fell ill, and called Dr. Rush. Keating eventually recovered, but the Irish Dominican and the German Bishop-elect were from the beginning almost hopeless cases. Rush on his sickbed feared he might lose "good Mr. Fleming the Roman priest" from not visiting him at his usual time. "The delay of a day, nay of a single hour, in administering the remedies proper in this disorder, is often fraught with irretrievable consequences," he observed. Whether for lack of more of Rush's bleedings, or for other cause, the "zealous and indefatigable" Father Fleming died on October 5, and Bishop Graessl followed him on the tenth. "He was my patient till the late return of my fever," Rush wrote of Graessl, "and I fear suffered from my being obliged to desert him."

The scholarly, affable Father Fleming and his distinguished German colleague were buried in the graveyard of St. Joseph's Church.

John Winkhause of the German Reformed and William Dougherty of the Methodist Church were both lost. Among Friends, fatalities exceeded four hundred. Daniel Offley, the merchant who joined the Committee and perished in his labors, had been a noted Quaker minister. So had Huson Langstroth, Michael Minier, and Charles Williams, all of whom died in Friendly service.

Altogether, ten of the preachers who remained in the city were victims of the plague—as many as doctors—and seven more at various times were desperately ill. The fever was undiscriminating. It granted no dispensation for faith, nor any for good works.

III

Philip Freneau, editor of the *National Gazette,* was having his troubles. They were more political than feverish. His cause —the cause of Citizen Genêt—was no longer an easy or popular one, for the French Minister had gone too far. Freneau resigned his clerkship in the State Department on October 11. He saw the collapse of his paper coming and prepared for that, too; but he held out through most of the plague, finally announcing the end of the *National Gazette* on October 27. Meanwhile he filled his columns with merry stuff calculated to cheer his desperate readers. His poem "Pestilence" made light of the whole epidemic; the death of a blacksmith gave him occasion for an "Elegy" filled with ridiculous puns:

> He blew up no coals of sedition, but still
> His bellows was always in blast;
> And we will acknowledge (deny it who will)
> That one Vice, and but one, he possessed.
>
> No actor was he, or concerned with the stage,
> No audience, to awe him, appeared;

Yet oft in his shop (like a crowd in a rage)
The voice of a hissing was heard.

Tho' steeling was certainly part of his cares,
In thieving he never was found;
And, tho' he was constantly beating on bars,
No vessel he e'er ran aground.

And the departure of the doctors, Shippen, Kuhn, and others,
Freneau celebrated in heroic verse, "Orlando's Flight":

On prancing steed, with spunge at nose,
From town behold Sangrado fly;
Camphor and Tar where'er he goes
Th' infected shafts of death defy—
    Safe in an atmosphere of scents,
    He leaves us to our own defence.

*   *   *   *

All this, and more, Sangrado knew,
(In Lucian is the story told)
Took horse—clapped spurs—and off he flew,
Leaving his Sick to fret and scold;
    Some soldiers, thus, to honour lost,
    In day of battle quit their post.

"The blessings of the poppy to relieve pain," the savagery
of country folk, the foolishness of fugitives, other tragedies of
the plague furnished fun in verse and dialogues for Freneau's
insensitive muse. He announced proudly that no employee of
the *National Gazette* caught the infection, which moved his
Federalist opponents to remark of course not, for Freneau was
immune—he had had a plague for years past. They advised him
to stop trifling with serious subjects, to renounce his infamy
and "endeavour to palm himself upon death for an honest man."

Freneau's finish as a political editor was at least one blessing
the Federalists could count when they returned to Philadelphia
after the fever.

IV

October 12, the managers reported, had been a very bad day
at Bush Hill. They had buried twenty-eight patients; the day

before, twenty. On the thirteenth, sixteen died. The Committee
at City Hall was likewise oppressed with the increase of deaths:
on October 11 they issued orders for twenty-four pauper inter-
ments; on the twelfth for twenty-nine, on the thirteenth for
twenty-one. Later, when all the figures had been gathered, these
charity patients were found to represent less than a quarter of
the daily victims. A note of despair began to creep into the
Committee's minutes. On October 17 Secretary Lownes made
the entry:

From the accounts received from different quarters of the city, it
is evident that the disorder now raging, has for the last week been
more general and alarming than at any time since its appearance—
its greatest height being about the 12th, the mortality at the Hospital also at that period, being greater than at any other time.

Two days later, the minutes recorded the only reference the
Committee made to the personal and human side of the plague:

Various instances of distress, some extremely afflicting, frequently occur, to enumerate them is difficult, such as have come
within the power of the committee to mitigate have been attended
to,—one of the carters in the service of the committee Reports,
that in the performance of his duty he heard the cry of a person in
great distress, the neighbours informed him, that the family had
been ill some days—and that being afraid of the disease no one had
ventured to examine the house; he cheerfully undertook the benevolent task, went up stairs and to his surprise found the father dead,
who had been lying on the floor for some days, two children near
him also dead, the mother in labour; he tarried with her, she was
delivered while he was there, and in a short time both she and her
infant expired! he came to the City Hall, took coffins and buried
them all.

For days, for weeks, Philadelphians had been hoping, waiting, praying for rain, under the impression that rain would
wash the air of its pestilence. Yet the weather remained mild
and warm. A rain finally came, pouring constantly, as Carey
wrote, during "the whole terrible twelfth of October, when one
hundred and eleven souls were summoned out of this world,
and a hundred and four the day following." This was the first
break in the drought since September 9; it was succeeded by

another storm on October 15, and these, Mayor Clarkson observed, brought cooler days in their wake, apparently checking the disorder, for the daily death rate fell to the eighties almost at once.

There it stayed, however, and disasters continued. James Wilson, the brave and conscientious Guardian of the Poor, on the fourteenth was himself admitted to Bush Hill where he had sent so many victims. Three days later he died. Jacob Tomkins, Jr., his colleague, was likewise carried off, and William Sansom was desperately ill, though eventually he recovered.

The business of the Guardians had been entirely assumed by the Committee, of necessity, for the demands of the sick and poor were greater than could be met with any but a large staff. Still more help was needed, however. There was a limit to what even an Israel Israel, a Samuel Benge could do. Simply to find all the starving was difficult, and to give them regular relief was a job for many workers. Accordingly, when the eight members of the Committee of Distribution were appointed (October 8) to receive applications for relief and provide for the poor, an "Assistant Committee" was also formed, "of respectable citizens, from the different parts of the city to recommend suitable objects for relief to the above committee of eight."

The Assistant Committee, formed thus in the height of the plague, marked the high point of the city's resistance to disaster. In September Clarkson had been able to persuade less than a score of people to devote themselves to relief. But so well had his small Committee functioned in three weeks, such examples had the twelve principal members set, that in October four dozen additional citizens were willing to come forward. Their help could not have been delayed longer, for with the stagnation of business, relief was required for hundreds of families ordinarily self-sustaining.

Samuel Coates, merchant—Rush described him as a very Anthony Benezet in the city's distress—was chairman of the assistants, and with John Oldden, merchant, as secretary set up headquarters in the crowded precincts of City Hall. The four dozen men worked under their direction. This constituted a sensible reorganization of the general Committee's work. The Assistant Committee became the arms, legs, eyes, and ears of those sitting at the City Hall with relief funds to spend. They went about the town collecting information, gathering victims, investigating needs, handing out relief certificates redeemable at City Hall.

The city was divided into ten districts, and each of the forty-six assistants prowled through his share of the deserted streets in search of distressed and stricken. The Northern Liberties and Southwark both made separate districts; in the city itself three men took the houses from the south side of Vine Street to the north side of Race, from river to river. Six others took Race to Arch, three Arch to Market, and so on, down to South Street, the southern edge. These long, narrow districts were difficult to handle, and included regions of great infection and slight; but at least they furnished an orderly method of administration. The forty-six volunteers were men of all ranks and stations, all churches and employments. They labored diligently at their dismal tasks. Carey observed that probably never before had so many indigent been relieved with so little imposition. Some persons in comfortable circumstances tried to secure relief on false representations, but these were detected. Many others really indigent would not deign to accept charity—these the assistants furnished with weekly loans, adequate for their immediate support, and took notes for the debt with no intention of demanding payment.

The assistants began their work on October 9. In a short while they were relieving as many as twelve hundred persons. On one day, 118 families were given money and provisions. On another, 112 families received one hundred dollars cash, more than twelve cords of wood, and a considerable supply of bread, meat, and vegetables. Still another day's report described the distribution of fifteen cords of wood, twenty dozen loaves of bread, meat, vegetables, and some fowls.

Even with utmost care, the assistants were not sure their

largesse was reaching all the needy. On October 25 Lownes, Carey, and Israel were appointed to meet with the assistants to provide "for such poor as may be suffering in obscurity." Next day Carey, Sharswood, and Lownes were directed to confer with the assistants regarding "suffering citizens whose modesty may prevent their obtaining that relief which their circumstances require." To persuade these diffident persons to accept loans, Thomas Savery and Samuel Benge were constituted a loan committee.

The Committee of Distribution was kept continually busy by the work of the assistants. The number of families daily relieved mounted above two hundred; Israel doled out cash, cordwood, chickens, turkeys, geese, bread, even sheep. Samuel Coates ran the business of the assistants with efficiency and firmness. He held frequent but brief general meetings at four in the afternoon in the upper front room of City Hall. When members failed in their duties for various reasons, all assistants were convened and new members at once appointed to replace them. When it was learned that the reports handed in were too general for the Committee of Distribution, Coates assembled his men and directed that every report "particularly state the number and condition of the family to be relieved, together with the exact sum of money, and specific kind of provisions as necessary for one week's subsistence." Coates, at the head of the assistants, was as firm and efficient as Mayor Clarkson in the general Committee.

The great quantity of provisions handed out by Israel's Committee of Distribution was the contribution of people outside Philadelphia to the plague-ridden city. As Philadelphians themselves had subscribed large sums in the past for the relief of disasters elsewhere, so now the citizens of other towns sent both money and goods to the capital. Boston raised $2,500, chartered the brig *Lark,* and sent her to Wilmington with 6,246 gallons of vinegar, 7,800 pounds of tallow candles, and 270 jugs of lemon juice for the stricken poor. New York's $5,000 came by cheque. Closer at hand, Germantown's committee raised $2,500 and authorized a further draft on themselves for as much as eight or even ten thousand dollars.

The delivery of donated goods into the city was a difficult feat, for even the most generous countryman or shipmaster had no wish to expose himself to contagion by entering the city. The Committee received numerous enquiries as to how the provisions might be delivered, from Montgomery, Bucks, and Berks, from Salem, Gloucester, and Haddonfield in Jersey and elsewhere. A Potts-Grove committee sent fourteen sheep and 106 fowl to Peter Robinson's mill, and later 212 more fowl. Henry Deforest found a wagon and sent it out to Robinson's to collect these provisions. Germantown inhabitants took their contributions as far toward the city as they dared. Peter Shiras of Mount Holly in Jersey actually came clear in to City Hall with £100 in his purse, but committees at Darby and Woodbury and in Delaware County asked for instructions for conveying their collections.

The Delaware County committee sent £200 to Nathaniel Newlin's house near Darby, and Deforest rode out to get it. Bridgetown, New Jersey, simply sent the cheques against Philadelphia correspondents to Wistar and Lownes. Some, like the committee of Franklin County and the Presbyterian congregation of Chestnut Level in Lancaster County, sent their monies to Governor Mifflin, inappropriately enough. Mifflin despatched General Proctor of the militia into City Hall with the funds. On other occasions, citizens or committeemen went to the wharves or the edge of the city to receive donations brought by persons who dared venture no further. Israel and Lownes one morning were called to the docks to receive from two members of the committee of Evesham Township, Burlington County, Jersey, $279.90, twenty-seven cheeses, twelve hams, and sundry other articles. The hams and cheeses were ordered sold and the proceeds laid out in articles "better adapted to the necessities of the poor." Later, Carey and Lownes met Isaac Lloyd at Weed's Ferry on the Schuylkill and received $1,448.21 from the residents of the Darby region. But the major part of the donations, the cords and flat loads of wood, the potatoes, flour, sheep, cheese, and fowl came in on carts or vessels, conveyed by haulers and packet-boat men at an exorbitant price.

The donations increased every day. Scarcely a township in the neighboring counties, scarcely a town, failed to send money or provisions or clothing or all three. As the weather cooled, firewood became vital. On October 16 John Haworth and Israel were named a committee to procure a supply of wood for Bush Hill and for the poor. They were "to continue to purchase, until they shall have 500 cords in store." For Israel Israel this additional duty was one too many, and at his request James Swain took his place. Actually, donations of wood came so rapidly that purchases were much less than expected. Straw was another favorite donation, particularly after October harvests. Dr. Robert Shannon of Norrington sent a hundred bundles, Benjamin Rittenhouse of Norristown another hundred. Milled flour also followed the harvest. Dr. Logan sent three cartloads of turnips from Stenton. Eggs, old linen, clothing, corn, vinegar, turkeys, chickens, and all manner of produce supplemented the gifts of money and credits. All were accompanied with letters of encouragement and good cheer.

The Bucks County Committee met at Newtown on October 19, with Henry Wynkoop in the chair. To the Philadelphia Committee Wynkoop wrote a long, elaborately constructed letter, begging that the Bucks County citizens be suffered "to share the honors of benevolence, and partake with you in the offices of social affection." Their distance from the dreadful scene not permitting any other aid than pecuniary, the committee which now addressed their Philadelphia friends had been formed, and had made such progress as to be able to assure one and all that their donations would do no discredit to their charitable dispositions. The Mayor's Committee had to pay the price of such eloquence to reap the benefits of Bucks nobility. The money collected waited only the direction of the Philadelphians, Wynkoop concluded:

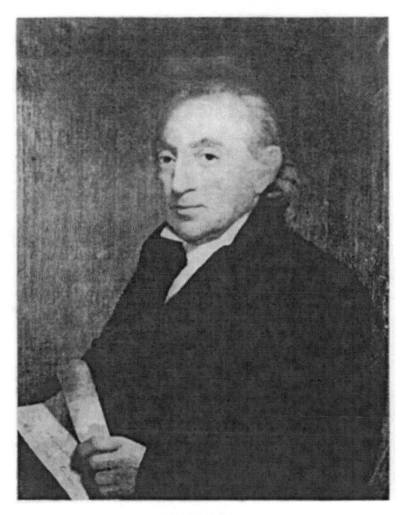

ISRAEL ISRAEL

What we wish principally at present is, that you would inform us of the place where, and the persons to whom you would wish the payments to be made; A letter therefore upon this head directed to the chairman of the committee will meet with due attention— In the mean time be assured that we are the friends of our fellow citizens, and particularly of those who are in distress: And may the great Ruler of the universe who ever chastens with the tenderness of a parent, look with compassion upon the sufferings of his children, and put a period to their afflictions—We remain worthy fellow citizens with esteem and sincerity,

Your friends and Humble Servants.

The busy Mayor's answer to this tiresome rhodomontade was not recorded.

v

Philadelphia these October days was the very caricature of a city, existence in it the very mockery of life. Everyone stayed indoors who could; one's next-door neighbor might die and be buried and those on all sides not know of it for days afterwards. Occasionally the foul odor of decaying flesh would inform neighbors and carters of a body behind closed doors and shuttered windows. Dust lay upon the streets as deep as two feet, grass turned brown, fire was a constant danger. The rains in the middle of the month brought some relief to the city, but came too late to help the farmers, whose crops failed in the drought.

This was the height of the plague, the height of demoralization, of despair, the height of disaster. The city was no human thing at all, but a place of quivering stench and filth, a place ruled by unreason. Everyone realized the uselessness of garlic, nitre, vinegar, tar, and camphor, but still they clung to their familiar nostrums from force of habit, took some comfort in their astringent smells. Every superstition, every homely legend, every traditional remedy was preserved, in all its ineffectualness. Tobacco was the universal preventive. Young Henry S. Drinker went out for a walk in Germantown with a segar in his mouth. He had never smoked before; the segar turned him to a green sweat. He staggered around to George Hesser's

orchard to discharge his stomach, fearful of doing so on the road
lest people suspect him of having the fever. Back in his mother's
parlor he was sick and pale.

And the cases, the fantastic tales of suffering, the separate
instances of death, piled one upon another in a great pyramid
of sorrow. Calamities multiplied beyond number. A man named
Collins buried his wife, two daughters, a son, his son's wife
and child; he married again, buried his new wife, and died himself. Samuel Shoemaker was thought to have died, and his
attendant went out to bring in a coffin. Returning, he found the
corpse sitting on the side of his bed putting on his shoes and
proposing to take a walk. The attendant objected, and begged
Shoemaker to lie down and rest. The good man did so, and died
a second time an hour later. Major David Franks, paymaster of
the Revolutionary army, loyal member of Philadelphia's synagogue, scion of a notable Jewish family of Montreal, sank quietly
into death alone in a hired room, under the care of a French
doctor. The carriers were about to bury him in Potter's Field
when honest John Thompson, a blacksmith with a wooden leg,
recognized his body and secured a grave for him in Christ
Church cemetery.

Cases, each different in detail, all alike in meaning, filled the
notebooks and mailboxes of the doctors. Old James Read, Esq.,
placeholder and bureaucrat, formerly prothonotary at Reading,
lived at 43 Newmarket Street in the Northern Liberties. Occasionally he went to the Admiralty office to do a little work, but
now a putrifying corpse lay in front of that office and no one
would remove it. Mr. Read stayed home with his daughter and
a faithful serving maid. He read the Christian fathers and his
Bible. Soon his daughter fell ill, and he called Dr. Rush. Then
for days upon days neither Rush nor anyone else came. Though
Read did not know it, Rush was lying helpless in his first bout
with the fever. On October 3 Read sent his ancient serving maid
to Third and Walnut with a note:

Dear, dear Doctor, Do come to see me—I am fatigued almost to
death—my precious Daughter is very, very weak—What can be the

Reason—no Citizen Doctor, or other Gent comes to see us. I am, Dr Sir, Yours ever affectionately, James Read. P.S. Your Medicine has wrought her almost to Death.

Rush could not go. He sent medicines, but next day Read wrote again. He himself had taken the fever, and his maid-servant was ailing.

Dear, very dear Friend: I beseech you come, *in Person* . . . My Daughter also wants you exceedingly, we don't know what to do— we beg, dear Sir, that you will come. . . . Your Physic wrought my child too much—I must be particular in my Direction, the Bearer being weak & apt to misunderstand.

By October 21 Read, his daughter, and the servant maid had all died, and were buried in a ditch that had been opened on the south side of Christ Church.

Cases among the doctors themselves mounted, too, with all their unsettling implications. Dr. Benjamin Say, when he recovered from his attack, took his wife and family down to Gray's Ferry. Here he had a country home, "The Cliffs," a red brick fortress whose towers overlooked the floating bridge and commanded a view of Bartram's Gardens across the Schuylkill. Mrs. Say was a Bonsall, a granddaughter of the botanist John Bartram who had planted the wonderland on the opposite bank. At The Cliffs, she caught the fever; so did her daughter, and both died. Dr. Say himself owed his life to the great purge, his friend Rush thought: twenty-three stools induced by calomel and gamboge had eliminated all the putrescence of his infection.

Dr. Currie's recovery Rush also attributed with vast irony to mercury and bleeding, for someone told him that Currie sank very low, and Dr. Hodge, who was treating him, in desperation actually resorted to Rush's cure. It was just one more example of the cowardly way his enemies would revile him, Rush explained to Timothy Pickering, yet secretly employ his method in their own illnesses. But Rush was misinformed. Hodge had treated Dr. Currie in his usual mild fashion, varying his system in one respect only—though an amazing one. He poured brandy down Dr. Currie in great quantities, and actually had the sick physician take a bath in brandy.

At the height, Rush estimated there were six thousand persons ill of the fever at once, with only three physicians able to be about. He was probably not far wrong in the number of cases, though he was clearly wrong in his notion that only three doctors were up and around. Rush was particular whom he called "physician."

All that they could learn the doctors garnered from each case, though now in October their observations were mixed with despair. Hemorrhages, Rush noted, occurred anywhere—in nose, gums, ears, stomach, bowels, urinary passages. Women's menses were remarkably copious, and came as much as two weeks early. The yellow color—that "golden yellow" as Currie called it, for which the disorder was named—Rush insisted rarely appeared when strong enough purges had been given; but when it did come it meant danger. It began first on the neck and breast; in one patient it commenced behind his ear and spread to the crown of his bald head. Rush knew some people mistrusted him because his patients did not show the yellow color of the fever in their faces. The answer was simple, he said; he put the yellowness "in a more suitable place by means of the strong, but safe mercurial purges."

And even in the height of the plague, even while he lay sick himself, Rush compiled his notes. He demanded every detail from his students, details of skin conditions, pimples, watery blisters, eruptions and scabs about the mouth, those little "petechiæ that resembled moscheto bites" on arms and breast, the carbuncles that discharged a thin, dark, bloody matter as in the true plague, every variety of skin disorder.

All his experience indicated that fear and grief caused a fever. And heat—bakers, blacksmiths, and hatters were particularly susceptible. And exercise—a long walk, a fall, or riding a hard-trotting horse were dangerous. And few who went gunning in the fields and marshes escaped the infection. Intemperance in drinking or eating invariably induced disease. Once a lady under

Dr. Mease's care came down following "a supper of sallad, dressed after the French fashion."

Patients could remain entirely conscious and in command of themselves, yet lose all memory of their days of sickness. Rush's pupil Fisher was perfectly composed and natural while the Doctor was treating him, yet on the sixth day when Rush took him by the hand and congratulated him on his recovery, he could recall nothing of what had passed in his room.

Rush continued to study the action of his medicine, noting with some dismay that it seemed to operate more slowly in October than it had in September. It had never succeeded without attendance and good nursing, but these were now seldom to be had. One of his patients, an elderly lady, died from lack of nursing, being attended only by a fourteen-year-old black child. The evacuating remedy could not work miracles.

It operated, however, under proper conditions. Rush found all the characteristics of bodies after death a proof of his analysis of the proximate cause, and of the effectiveness of his medicine. He described these post-mortem facts with great care. Most bodies turned yellow a few minutes after death, though some became purple or black. Soberly, he recorded one body yellow above the waist and black below. Stiffness was always sudden, coming in one to six hours. Many bodies discharged blood and black matter from bowels, nose, and mouth immediately after death—so abundantly as to require lining the coffins in which all were buried with a heavy pitch.

But, Rush remarked, the science of medicine was related to everything, and as he made his rounds through the city he was as much interested to observe the minds and manners of people as the details of medical practice. Dr. Rush was part of a general, instinctive conspiracy to ignore the rioting and lewdness in the city. Only occasionally, even in Brown's *Federal Gazette,* did anyone refer to misconduct and vice that all observed. Sailors were blamed for much of it (a Philadelphia habit). Seamen's taverns below the drawbridge were described as hotbeds of crime, and on the waterfront high prices were bid for goods landed by seamen without the formalities of customs examination. Joshua Dawson of the Treasury wrote of "fine doings in the River, easy means of smuggling, & most likely, little precaution taken to prevent it."

Rush was loath to record any irregularities. The moral senses, he declared in one place, were actually improved by the city's disasters. But elsewhere he was more truthful, recording that convalescence was marked "by a sudden revival of the venereal appetite" which occasioned numerous weddings, twelve among the patients recovering at Bush Hill. "I wish I could add," he confessed, "that the passion of the sexes for each other, among those subjects of public charity, was always gratified only in a lawful way. Delicacy forbids a detail of the scenes of debauchery which were practised near the hospital, in some of the tents which had been appropriated for the reception of convalescents."

Yet the "morbid excitability of the venereal appetite" was not so great in Philadelphia as it had been in Messina in 1743, he added, comfortably.

VI

At the height of the plague, Philadelphia's institutions fell to pieces. The Pennsylvania Hospital Board of Managers, like the College of Physicians, had to give up their regular meetings; they agreed that any manager who could should attend the hospital as often as his health would permit, and asked Rush and Parke (the only remaining hospital doctors) to walk the wards, Wistar to consult with them as a favor. The Post Office was in complete disorder, letters neither sent nor delivered; every day a vinegared crowd of people lined up at the University to get mail. The Library Company closed. The directors had failed to meet in September; only Benjamin Poultney turned up. By October Poultney was dead, and no other directors were in town.

The city recorder decamped, and John Donaldson, Register General of Public Documents, was obliged to report to the Governor that "the present deranged state of the Officers of accounts occasioned by the malignant Fever" made it impossible to draw certificates for the regular quarterly salary due to government officials. Most of the "deranged" officials, busy with their safety, scarcely minded the absence of their pay cheques, but the Sixth Company of Artillery, on duty at Fort Mifflin, was not so complacent. Captain Woodside demanded immediate payment for his men. He did agree at the Governor's urging, however, to forbear prosecuting a duel to which he had challenged Lieutenant Thompson, both because of the calamitous state of the city, and because Thompson had just lost his wife in the fever.

And as institutions, so men decayed. The spirit of fellowship, the dignity and humanity of men, disappeared in the struggle to survive. What fear had wrought in September, hopeless despair reproduced in October. Landlords, rapacious and unpitying, foreclosed and evicted without regard to the condition of renters. A wealthy widow secured from the Committee of Distribution grants of money for several of her tenants as worthy objects of relief, but she promptly appropriated the money, seized the clothing of her tenants, and turned them out. One man lost his wife and came down with the fever himself; he recovered blind, penniless, burdened with two small children, yet even before he could leave his sickbed his landlord seized his furniture and clothes and evicted him.

Negro nurses were beset with strange requests. People in full health would ask Jones, Gray, or Allen to promise to care for them in sickness, and would arrange for their burial in advance. Some even lay on the floor to be measured for their coffins. A fatalism, a despondency, a certainty of death gripped the imagination of hundreds. Reality was even worse. Many died alone, unseen and unassisted. The colored carriers found them

in various situations, some laying on the floor, as bloody as if they had been dipt in it, without any appearance of their having had even a drink of water for their relief ; others laying on a bed with their clothes on, as if they had come in fatigued, and lain down to rest ; some appeared, as if they had fallen dead on the floor, from the position we found them in.

After the Negroes began to bleed following Rush's directions they learned still more about human nature. Sometimes, they observed, a patient would declare he was much improved as soon as he felt the prick of the knife. From these the nurses took blood copiously. Others were completely indifferent and lethargic, and those the Negroes learned to bleed sparingly. Continually, intimately exposed, Negroes sickened in great numbers; more than three hundred perished in the plague.

All who went from house to house, midwives, barbers, hairdressers, even bleeders, were shunned. Some citizens bought their own lancets in order to be free of dependence upon commercial leeches. Numerous churches were deserted, and Friends' Yearly Meeting adjourned after a sparsely attended session. Other churches, however, continued to hold services, and sharp controversy arose over the wisdom of collective piety at such a time.

Half the servants of the city deserted their masters (small wonder, Rush thought). The gravediggers in Potter's Field worked on shifts around the clock, and a tent was set up in the field to accommodate them in their short hours of rest. "Not a ray of alleviation of the present calamity breaks in our city from any quarter," Rush wrote Julia. "All is a thick and melancholy gloom." At John Meredith's store the Doctor picked up a little baby, who lay smiling and crowing in his arms, innocently happy in the midst of horror. "All hearts now are faint, and all hope is in God alone."

Yet curiously, even in these worst days of all, there were enterprising spirits. One of the Santo Domingans, Louis F. R. A. Gatereau, chose the height of the plague to commence publishing his *Courrier Politique de la France et de ses Colonies,* a triweekly newspaper printed at John Parker's establishment in Second Street. And Tanguy de la Boissiere, one of the ablest of the Haitians, brought his paper *Journal des Revolutions de la Partie Française de Saint-Domingue* down from New York just before the beginning of October. Somehow, serene spirits like Tanguy and Gatereau seemed immune from the fever. Dr. Isaac

Cathrall (himself the jolliest of men) remarked, as did Rush and others, that the cheerful, fearless, and gay, the idiots and maniacs, escaped infection.

And in the worst of the plague the regular fall general election was held. Past the coffins, the crowds, the smoking tar barrels around the State House filed a few of the electors from the city and near-by townships. The usual accompaniments of an election were absent—the speeches, the ale, the crowds, the rivalry. Before the fever began it had been said that Mifflin would have a very close race, that Muhlenberg had a good chance of beating him. But with the light vote in Philadelphia there was really no contest. Mifflin and his party won easily through the whole state, by a 2-1 margin of the votes cast. The plague had spared the easy-going Governor even the trouble of a campaign.

And for those who looked without prejudice, French medicine offered hope. Dr. Griffitts, who spoke French fluently, was amazed at the apparent success of methods he disapproved of. Had he bothered to consult with the French doctor Nassy he might have doubted the correctness of Rush's theories. Dr. Nassy visited 160 patients from August 28 to October 10; 117 of them had the yellow fever, he lost only nineteen. Of these nineteen, eleven he had seen only on the second, fourth, or fifth day, after other physicians had treated them with the violent Rushite medicines.

And throughout the height of the plague, as the October moon rode high over devastation and people prayed for release, a sense of normality was preserved by the regular appearance of Andrew Brown's *Federal Gazette*. Every day it came on the streets on schedule, to record the thin trickle of trade in the city, and to circulate the latest opinions of the fever. Brown had no easy time of it. Printers fled or sickened, supplies ran short, deliveries were difficult. The paper on which he printed was made at mills near Wilmington, and neither vessels nor carts would bring it up. Twice in September and again for nine days in October he was obliged to print on half-sheets.

Financial problems plagued him as soon as business houses began to close. He kept his advertising columns filled out with notices which should have been "killed" long before—July and August arrivals, sales, runaways, departures. He republished his original statement of the "plan and conditions" of the *Gazette,* republished it several times, for it filled a whole column, and the type he always held standing anyway. He printed other columns of undistributed type, such as the Governor's proclamations of the previous April, and miscellaneous city ordinances. Sometimes whole pages of such dead filler stuff would appear. These produced no revenue. Had it not been for chemists' advertisements of bark, vinegar, and purges, he must have failed —those, and legal notices of decedents' estates. All who had claims against the late Jacob Tryon, tinplate-worker, or Richard Hicks, parchment- and glue-maker, or William Stiles, stone-cutter, or scores of others were advised to make immediate demand. Such notices were set in the same stick with the offerings of Dr. Rush's Mercurial Sweating Powders faithfully prepared by various druggists, appeals for the return of runaway slaves and servants, advertisements of houses for sale or let.

October 1 was the birthday of the *Federal Gazette*—its fifth— and Brown followed his custom of addressing his readers in a publisher's letter. He was determined to proceed, he announced, however great the difficulties. In such a critical period a distressed city needed its newspapers more than ever, and his had become the only daily means of communicating information generally. From every quarter of the Union he learned that the continuation of his paper "amid scenes of uncommon danger and of daily threatening mortality" had been of great use to the people. "It has kept whole the chain of general intelligence that must otherwise have been broken," he wrote. And, being a just man, he printed a tribute to one of his apprentices, a boy who never missed a day's work, who delivered papers the whole length of Water Street and was never known to complain.

Columns of "European Intelligence," correspondence "By This Day's Mail," essays on public issues by various ancient

Romans which Brown clipped from such other American papers as he could procure, were like windows opening to a fresh, familiar landscape for Philadelphia readers, isolated in their gloomy loneliness. And the local columns, both paid and free, were a mirror held to the city, a picture of the plague year drawn by the people themselves. Lost dogs, stray horses, runaway slaves American and Santo Domingan, escaped prisoners, fugitive apprentices, disappearing servants, all found their way to the *Gazette*. Property of the dead was put up for sale, young men out of work solicited positions, proprietors out of help offered jobs. Wet-nurses and bartenders were wanted universally, at high pay.

When Citizen Robert came from Boston, Brown gave half a column to his credentials and nobility of soul; but quacks and empirics had to buy their public notices. Dr. Chambard, *Chirurgien François,* lately arrived, paid to advertise in French and English that he could be of service to those afflicted with disorders incident to human nature: without drugs, with only the simplest herbs, he could cure the flux, the inveterate itch, ulcers, venereal disease, rheumatism, gravel, hysterics, and fever; and mercury lodged in the bones from former prescriptions he could eliminate by the methods of nature. M. Courbé, actually a qualified Santo Domingan doctor, contented himself with a simple professional card; but a Mr. Mahy took four column inches to describe a wonderful and unique English Powder he had for sale at $2 a dose. And a certain Samuel Correy offered at the City Hall, for no fee whatsoever, a medicine costing three shillings ninepence, procurable at any druggist's, which was a speedy and efficacious cure for the yellow spotted fever. As a bonus to this generous gift, he supplied a prescription (gin, honey, and a corrosive sublimate) by which nurses could render themselves immune. Correy was a source of embarrassment to Brown. He boldly used Dr. Physick's and Dr. Cathrall's names as references for his wonderful cure, and Brown was obliged to give the young physicians space for letters denying any acquaintance with the quack or his nostrums.

To bona fide medical testimony and argument, Brown gave
most of his local news space. Letters of Dr. Mease and Dr.
Griffitts describing their own bleedings at Rush's hand and
their faith in the great evacuating remedy, as well as letters
from laymen bearing grateful witness to the success of Rush
in their cases, Brown knew had both local and general appeal.
He ran them, along with Rush's own letters to John Rodgers
and other smaller pieces the Doctor indited from his sickbed to
prove his theories and the errors of his opponents. But Brown
was too earnest a man, and too wise a publisher to take sides.
With professions of impartiality, he likewise published the letters of Wistar, Ruston, all the others, and of those who objected
to the whole medical controversy. The news of other cities'
donations was daily fare by mid-October, replacing former stories of their cruelty and injustice. Essays comparing the French
mode of diet and dress with the American, religious exhorta-
tions and ascriptions of the pestilence to divine anger, took
column after column, and plenty of correspondents had barbed
comments for fugitive citizens. To these last, Brown himself
replied, in an article praising the worthy Mayor and the gentlemen of the Committee but begging that fugitives, except doctors
and ministers, be not condemned, asking only that those who
fled remember all they owed to those heroic ones who led the
city in its trials.

Obituaries Brown published sparingly, and with curious randomness. Several times he devoted a whole stick to obscure
but pious people, while civic leaders received only a few lines;
but Samuel Johnson, printer and bookseller, president of the
printers' Franklin Society, was accorded a half-column by his
fellow artisan. Of the ten doctors who died, Hutchinson was
singled out for lavish praise, Graham was adequately lamented,
but the others were passed over with a word. Brown obviously
had no wish to burden his readers with necrology. Instead, he
gave always what consolation he could find, even inserting once
(October 2) a ribald satire on the whole plague picture.

Satires were welcome relief, particularly after Freneau's *Na-*

tional Gazette began its death rattle. Brown's satire was a
Dialogue between two Jersey farmers, William and George,
which ridiculed the fears of country people about coming into
the city. William wished to go to market, and knew George had
just returned. He consulted him about the danger. Only the
high prices for his produce had induced him to go, George
confessed. He had stopped all the openings of his body—the
two lower with a tight cork and a strong leather string, his nose
and ears with putty, his mouth with a large handkerchief. From
Cooper's Ferry (Camden) he could see the fever, clear across
the river. The city was as yellow as a pumpkin patch, and as he
walked down Water Street he was suddenly struck by such a
fog of smell pouring forth from a house in which fifty-nine
people had died that he was knocked clear across the street, and
lay sprawling in the gutter. The fever killed stone dead in a
moment. In a few minutes in town, he saw six fall without warning. But feeling a chill pass over him instead of heat, he knew
he was still safe. He went at once to the market, where he received five shillings ninepence for his butter, four shillings for
eggs. Only his inability to hear or speak through his various
protective gags prevented him getting more. He learned that
14,200 had died, that 29,000 had fled, and only 1,425 people
were left in the city.

Yet—five and nine for butter, four shillings for eggs! cried
William. He would risk it, at all hazards, on the morrow—
and if he returned would tell George of his own adventures!

Frost

*... the Great Disposer of winds and rains, took his
own time, and without the means, either moral or
physical, on which we placed our chief reliance, to
rescue the remnant of us from destruction.*
                                        —MATHEW CAREY

GENERAL WASHINGTON, from the placid scenes of Mount
Vernon, began writing some puzzled letters around the first of
October. The government was in ridiculous confusion, with
clerks and secretaries scattered all over the country; the President was receiving letters that should have gone to underlings.
And no one seemed to know where the official papers and records were. General Washington had a profound respect for
public papers. He liked all files kept neatly and in order, so he
could know in a moment everything that was going on. But
now, with the new Congress scheduled to meet in December,
no work was being done, and most of those who should be
working were not even to be found.

Everyone told Washington the fever in Philadelphia was
growing worse. Not that his sources of information were very
reliable—of all the government, only Randolph, Pickering, and
Wolcott were left near the capital city, and they did not write
him regularly. He heard from two colonels who had it from
a man who had it from Governor Mifflin that Mayor Clarkson
was reported to have said that more than 3,500 had died. Another report put the dead above four thousand and included
Thomas Willing, Jonathan Dickinson Sergeant, and Colonel
Franks among the victims. But Washington wanted accurate,
reliable news. Not to be informed was embarrassing. "It is a

delicate situation for the President to be placed in," he complained.

It became more delicate as October wore on. Congress had to meet, not only to deal with the French question, but also to take some sensible measures about the public offices and papers. Yet congressmen could not come to the plague center, and how could they constitutionally be called together anywhere else? Certainly the President had no power to change the capital of the nation.

General Washington was scrupulous on constitutional matters. He talked with Jefferson, who gave little help. Neither the constitution nor the laws empowered the President to change the place where Congress was to meet, Jefferson said. Washington feared as much. He began seeking advice. "I wish to hear the opinions of my friends upon all difficult and delicate subjects," he explained. To Randolph, Wolcott, and Pickering, to Hamilton, Knox, and Jefferson, to Congressman James Madison and Speaker of the House Trumbull, he appealed. Did the executive have power to convene Congress anywhere he chose, in case of emergency? If so, what place should he choose?

Washington's own preference was for Germantown. That would show no sectional partiality, and would leave the Congress free to move back to Philadelphia when health was restored. He resolved to gather the Cabinet at Germantown on November 1, and asked Randolph to procure hired lodgings for him, or quarters at "one of the most decent Inns."

Meanwhile answers to his puzzle began coming in. Well-meaning citizens sent or published letters to him, headed "Where will Congress meet?" Hamilton, whom he had prayed to "dilate fully" upon the constitutional issue, was more encouraging than Jefferson. Of course the President could change the place of Congress' meeting, Hamilton wrote. It was entirely within the Constitution. The capital city might be taken by an enemy army, or swallowed up by an earthquake, just as now it was devastated by fever. But this certainly did not mean that government must cease.

Yet Jefferson still said otherwise, and Madison agreed with him. The Constitution, these friends advised General Washington, used "particular caution" to avoid giving the President power over the place of meeting, lest he exercise it "with local partialities." The residence law said Philadelphia was to be the capital until the year 1800, when the new federal city on the Potomac would be ready. And all the executive officers should now get as close to the capital as possible. As for Congress, where they met was up to the members; but Jefferson and Madison thought they were obliged to come together in Philadelphia according to adjournment, "even if it be in the open fields," before they moved elsewhere by their own action.

Attorney-General Randolph agreed with Jefferson. The President could not move Congress. "It seems to be unconstitutional," Randolph said. The thing to do was to assemble the executive department somewhere, then let the congressmen meet at their constitutional time within the bounds of Philadelphia, and decide for themselves where to go.

But where should the President wait for them? The executive had to be available to Congress when the session was ready for work. Pickering said simply, Go to Germantown. Though it was crowded now, the Postmaster-General wrote, many Philadelphians would return home by December 2, the meeting day of Congress, for Dr. Rush assured him that long before December the fever would have ceased. And besides, leading Philadelphia citizens expected Congress to come back as though nothing had happened. Oliver Wolcott said the same thing, and urged Germantown.

But Randolph said Germantown could not possibly accommodate the Congress. It was a good enough place for the Cabinet to meet and decide on further measures, but far too small to house the whole government. Governor Mifflin, he wrote, intended convening the Pennsylvania Assembly there at the same time. The few large houses and seven inns around the village would be packed with Pennsylvanians. Foreign ministers and consuls would have to live in "dirty hovels," and all the government would be unhappy, because in Germantown there was not a single church of the English language.

Randolph thought Lancaster would be the best place. (He had just sent his family there.) He advised against Reading: Judge Rush, who lived there, said Reading had no accommodations. Yet Colonel Pickering had come through Reading in the summer and he thought Judge Rush was wrong. The government could exist, though not comfortably, in the courthouses and the various dwellings in the little town. President Washington had already decided against Wilmington and Trenton, for they were on main highways from Philadelphia and therefore dangerous. And to go as far south as Annapolis, or north as New York, would arouse all the sectional jealousies that had split the Congress at the time of the Residence Act.

Washington was in a quandary. He asked Madison and Randolph both to draft some instrument he could use to tell Congress officially where he was, one that might perhaps persuade the two houses to join him. Then, not quite sure what would happen, he announced that he would go to Germantown at the end of the month.

The fever, he heard, was finally abating. Pickering wrote on October 21 that it was reduced at least one-half. For days, Pickering wrote, Dr. Rush had been thronged with applicants, but on the twenty-first he spent the whole day at the Doctor's, and not one new patient sent for advice. Dr. Devèze, moreover, said only three cases at Bush Hill were in a dangerous state. Or so Pickering heard, anyway.

But Wolcott warned the President not to come soon. Around October 15 the weather had been cool, and rain with several frosty nights had greatly diminished the disease. But warmer days succeeded, Wolcott wrote, and brought a recurrence of cases. On the twentieth he was still apprehensive. The town was not yet safe, and would not be for days to come.

Washington decided to leave his family at Mount Vernon. With only his secretary, a coachman, and a valet, he left home on October 28 and rode northward. At Baltimore he met

Thomas Jefferson, who came in all alone on the Fredericksburg stage.

No coach lines were running north of Baltimore. The President and the Secretary of State had to hire a private carriage, and through Elkton, Wilmington, and on to Germantown were exposed to every inconvenience known to travel. Heat, cold, dust, and rain, the extortion of ferrymen and the rapacity of landlords—Jefferson complained of them all. The President serenely ignored hardships, but Jefferson inveighed against the "harpies who prey upon travellers," computing that the whole journey cost him nearly eighty dollars. And when they reached Germantown on Friday, November 1, Washington could go to the comfortable house of the Reverend Frederick Herman, where Randolph had arranged lodging for him, but Jefferson, at the King of Prussia tavern, could obtain nothing better than a bed in the corner of a public room. Even that was "a great favor," he observed. The only other choice was to sleep in his greatcoat before the fire.

What annoyed Jefferson most was that Philadelphians would not take courage enough to go home, thus vacating rooms in the King of Prussia. The house was so crowded that prices soared beyond reason. "We must give from 4 to 6 to 8 dollars a week for cuddies without a bed, and sometimes without a chair or table," he wrote indignantly. But he engaged beds for Madison and Monroe in the public room, and advised them to join him.

President Washington, meanwhile, quietly settled down to work, after his efficient fashion. In Mr. Herman's study he began his endless correspondence the very evening he arrived. Interminable reading and writing had been the heart of his public life for twenty years.

II

Plagues do not end with dramatic suddenness. They taper off. Cold weather comes, mosquitoes die, birds go south; by and by there are no more sudden seizures, someone says the pestilence is over. Deaths continue, people grow bold and care-less, there is needless waste of life. But the terror ceases. Many wonder what they feared, or what resisted. Such were the last days of October.

It is not deaths that make a plague, it is fear and hopelessness in people. Now, even though daily death rates persisted at a level higher than any week in August, fear and hopelessness were conquered. Purifying winter was coming on. Clear, sharp fall air was air to breathe deep and be joyous in, not foul, putrid, damp and sticky stuff full of mysterious solids and infectious fluids. Philadelphians could see the light ahead. They were on the way out of their cave of sorrows.

Each October day everyone counted the deaths, and watched the weather. Rains would surely purge the aether of its mi-asmata—rains, thunder, lightnings, and wind. So when the heavy rains of Saturday October 12, came, the whole city breathed easier, looked gratefully to the lowering sky. But that day 111 died.

Sunday was fair and cool; it was expected to be worse, yet only 103 died. And though Monday was calm, warm, and dry, still the toll dropped, to eighty-one. Oddly, the old belief that rains and cold killed the fever, warm and dry weather fostered it, seemed wrong.

For three days, October 15 to 18, deaths stood around eighty. Then they suddenly dropped still lower, to sixty, and stayed there four days, though skies were clear. The temperature fell once to 41 degrees; it rose no higher than 66.

Sixty deaths a day meant a reduction by half. Rush, Clarkson, all who studied the figures, were convinced on Monday, Octo-ber 21, that the end was finally in sight.

But on Tuesday the twenty-second eighty-two died.

It was hard to make sense out of these figures. People who remembered the plague of 1762 knew that it had ended with the frost. But only now were they recalling how long it took to end, how many days it hung on after the weather had changed, how many died in the last days of the fever. The drop in deaths to half of their peak figure was only a statistic. It did not cure those who were still infected, nor did it erase the infection. Fever lurked everywhere—around corners, in closed houses, in swamps and fields. The cause still existed, Oliver Wolcott wrote, and as long as the cause was there, no one could be safe.

Curiously, the fever seemed to migrate. It moved out of the very heart of town, where it had taken so many lives, and into the suburbs—to Southwark, the Northern Liberties, Frankford, "other out parts." Cooler weather appeared to do nothing but spread the infection.

To those who had endured twelve weeks of misery, living only for the time when winter would dissolve their torture, this disappointment destroyed all hope. Even snow and sleet would not remove the infection, some said. Many fugitives resolved never to go back to Philadelphia.

Joshua Dawson, Treasury clerk, saw young Mr. Laurence in Hamilton's office die on October 15, Mathew Walker of the register's office on the eighteenth. Yet he was told on the nineteenth that the plague diminished greatly, and that Secretary Hamilton was on his way back to town. On the twenty-first he described a general "abatement." Dr. Wistar assured him the disease was no longer violent, or alarming in appearance.

But when Tuesday the twenty-second brought its eighty-two deaths, for no reason, all Dawson's old alarm returned. Why, he wondered, were deaths always greater on Monday and Tuesday than the rest of the week? Perhaps the crowded congregations on Sunday evenings carried the fever.

On Wednesday the twenty-third the thermometer stayed down in the fifties. A high wind blew from the west. When the day was over, only fifty-four had died. Thursday took only thirty-eight, Friday thirty-five, Saturday twenty-three. The week ended hopefully, though Southwark was still full of patients. On Sunday only thirteen died. It turned cold that night, and Monday the twenty-eighth began with a light frost. But on Monday twenty-four were buried. Every time people glimpsed the end, daily tolls in this manner would jump up again.

Yet the drop from over a hundred to a mere two dozen deaths a day was an unmistakable sign that the end was near. Why, no one knew. Those who said weather had something to do with it were clearly refuted by the facts, Mathew Carey observed. He tabulated temperatures, barometric readings, and daily deaths, to prove that whatever caused the abatement, it was not weather. "In fact," he added, "the whole of the disorder, from its first appearance to its final close, has set human wisdom and calculation at defiance."

Yet, if no one understood, at least all could recognize, that the terror and dread were over. First to sense it were the members of the Committee. Samuel Benge found fewer burials every day, the managers at Bush Hill received fewer patients; now they were sending more to the convalescent home than to the graveyard. The assistants, walking up and down their districts, discovered no new victims. Instead, people were coming out of hiding, opening their houses, even going out of doors.

On Saturday, October 26, the Committee found their business a lighter burden than they had known in the whole forty days of their existence. They listened to encouraging reports: only twelve admissions at Bush Hill, only two deaths; no burials at all by Samuel Benge. The appearance of things, they resolved, "afforded much consolation."

Accordingly the Committee prepared an announcement, addressed to "their fellow citizens throughout the United States": the disorder abated beyond all expectation, soon it would be gone entirely. No one should return for a week or ten days, however, "or until there shall be a considerable fall of rain; as the change of air might prove dangerous, and probably fatal to many."

Then the members, looking at one another in relief and sympathy, passed another resolution, a purely personal one, which more than anything else signalized their relief:

It having pleased Divine Providence to favor us with an agreeable prospect of returning health to our long afflicted city—And as several of the members of the committee are desirous of attending their respective places of worship, it is Agreed, that those who have no indispensable duties to perform at the City Hall, be at liberty to withdraw their attendance to morrow.

It was the first Sunday since September 15 that they had thought of going to church.

Dr. Rush, like the Committee, began to relax. He even made plans for the future. To see his beloved wife again, to see all his children, appeared now a possibility. On the twenty-first he left his house and went about the city for the first time since his illness. More people were in the streets, he noticed, and they no longer wore a hangdog look. But next day came that sudden revival of deaths. "O! that God would hear the cries and groans of the many hundred, perhaps thousand sick which still ascend to his throne every hour of the day and night, from our desolating city!" Rush wrote. He felt their plight all the more, enfeebled as he was, unable to help them. And he heard constantly of patients "being murdered by large and ill-timed doses of bark and wine."

Dr. Sproat's son-in-law was being treated by Dr. Hodge. He was therefore doomed, Rush thought. For Hodge he still had nothing but resentment. "It is truly distressing to think of the desolation which has followed the footsteps of this man," he exclaimed.

Yet on the twenty-fourth only half a dozen people came to see Rush, and by the twenty-sixth he could write that his whole neighborhood was pure—not a single sick person within a square of Third and Walnut.

Rush found time for other matters, for finances particularly. He had sent out no bills during the pestilence; he had actually spent more than £200 in coach rentals, services, all the needs of his busy days. His clothes were so ragged he was ashamed of them. Yet William Hamilton, his landlord, the laird of Bush Hill, raised his rent, and sent a note demanding payment for the quarter. Rush was deeply hurt at such insensitivity. He determined to move, as soon as Julia could come back.

By the twenty-eighth, Rush was still living in "so small a sphere" that he knew little of affairs in the city, but he wrote confidently that "the disease visibly and universally declines." He began to purify his house. The whole family moved into the front parlor. "Our little back parlour has resembled for two months the cabin of a ship," he wrote. "It has been shop, library, council chamber, dining room, and at night a bed chamber for one of the servants." Now his mother hired a cook to relieve Marcus, and the colored servant (with the help of little Peter, who was peevish and cross, but recovered) began to whitewash the rooms and soak the furniture in vinegar.

All over the city, fugitives were coming back by October 21. Shutters banged back on houses, windows were thrown up. The fugitives made a strange contrast to those who had stayed. They were fat, healthy, ruddy, frequently they smiled. They found their friends changed sometimes beyond all recognition. Everyone in the city was gray with fatigue, gaunt and haggard, yellow with the jaundice of disease. Those who had taken the mercury spat continually, their teeth were black.

The fugitives found Philadelphia streets cleaner, neater, emptier than they had ever known them. No beggars, no orphan children, no poor lay in the alleys; no waste of the markets or refuse of commerce blocked the way.

Suddenly the fever seized some of the returned fugitives. Immediately the Committee published a warning: Let all those returning take every precaution, air their houses completely for several days, burn nitre to purge the foul solids from the aether, throw quicklime in their privies, whitewash all bedrooms where sick had been.

But workmen were now as scarce as nurses. To hire whitewashing was nearly impossible. All available painters and carpenters were engaged by those who were building or remodeling, or for government projects like the roofing of Congress Hall.

Joshua Dawson undertook to have all the Treasury offices thoroughly cleansed; the expense was enormous, but it had to be done. And the merchant John Welsh bid high for laborers before he could persuade any to clean his home and warehouse.

By October 25 boats began coming up from Wilmington and Chester, stores began to open, tradesmen appeared on the docks. And on Saturday the twenty-sixth country people flocking in to the market found it plentifully provisioned and fully attended for the first time. Butchers stood to their blocks again, blood ran once more in the gutters, sheep's heads rolled in the stalls. Twenty-three died in the city that day, but they had been a long time sick.

All the last week of October deaths remained about twenty a day, but the optimism of the people was irrepressible. Andrew Brown wrote a paragraph on the "dawn of returning health and order." Lottery drawings were advertised; Mrs. Scott, midwife, announced her return to the city; Rayner Taylor was printing "an anthem suitable to the present occasion." The stage lines informed the citizens they would resume normal operation on November 4. Public offices would be opened as soon as they could be fumigated, cleaned, and whitewashed. The new city auctioneer, appointed in the room of Adam Hubley, who had died, would commence business as soon as he could procure a store, "and the present melancholy times admit."

Columns were filled with advertisements for creditors of decedents' estate, clerks advertised for jobs, merchants for clerks, and anyone who wanted his mail delivered at home, as formerly, was directed to tell the postmaster.

On the last day of October the managers thought to make an effect. They hoisted over Bush Hill a huge white flag with the legend clearly legible far off, "No More Sick Persons Here." But it was too soon. True enough, Benge had taken no one out to the lazaretto that day, but on November 1 two new patients came in, on the second, two; on the third, four. The flag had to be hauled down. The fever was going to last into November.

The Committee knew a week of tense waiting. More orphans

were discovered, Benge still had two or three dead each day; but Bush Hill was able to report that two men buried on the sixth were the first dead in five days.

Now clearly the malignant fever was gone, but just as clearly there were as many deaths the first week in November as there had been that last week in August when the College of Physicians had met and precipitated the general alarm. They rose once above twenty, even though the temperature was below freezing, and they were still at fifteen on the eighth. And there were new cases. Mr. Brooks, the silversmith, had come back to town on October 31. He caught the fever, died on November 3.

The Committee, observing the deaths, published a warning. The disorder abated, and would doubtless soon be gone, but it had not disappeared yet. It still lurked in different parts of the city. The unsettled weather, the sudden cold, was unhealthy. Let those still in the country stay yet awhile; let those returned purify their houses instantly, or the Committee would have to do it for them.

But citizens who had once failed to take precautions from fear now failed from indifference. Nothing had stopped panic in September; nothing could stop optimism in November. Nor did anyone wish to. Stephen Girard, whose daily reports had so long been grim and terse, now came close to making a joke. On November 4 he reported that four persons had died, "to wit: a young man of the fever, a woman of a dropsy, one by a miscarriage, and one of old age."

When Girard could speak like this of his grim business, the fever was truly disappearing.

III

The last of October found Benjamin Rush in a reflective mood. He was still weak, he made no calls, he only stayed in town to encourage and advise Fisher and Coxe. Most of his time he spent reading, or making notes on the epidemic.

Sometimes seated in your easy chair by the fire [he wrote Julia], I lose myself in looking back upon the ocean which I have passed, and now and then find myself surprised by a tear in reflecting upon the friends I have lost, and the scenes of distress that I have witnessed, and which I was unable to relieve.

He remembered those awful days in August—it seemed years ago—when he had not yet discovered his cure.

I viewed a corner of the front room in which I sat in silence and darkness for half an hour, at a time when the disease baffled the power of medicine. I felt over again all the horror and distress wch. the prospect of the almost, or perhaps total desolation of our city at that time excited in my mind. I cast a look (I then thought, most probably a final one) towards my dear family, for I had resolved to perish with my fellow citizens rather than dishonor my profession or religion by abandoning the city. I can never forget the anguish of soul with which in this awful situation I wrung my hands, and I believe I wept aloud.

Now it was only a memory, however, a retrospect of past troubles. He opened his Bible as he finished his letter to his wife. *"The winter is gone,"* he wrote, *"the flowers appear upon the earth, the time of the singing of birds is come, and the voice of the turtle is again heard in our land."*

Even in his weakness, Rush was not through fighting. He found many Philadelphians turned against him because he said the fever originated locally. Such a view would destroy the city's reputation for healthiness, hurt commerce, drive Congress away. But Rush persisted. "Truth in science as morals never did any harm," he declared.

Tench Coxe, commissioner of the revenue, wrote John Adams the first week in November that two of the fugitive physicians had returned, the Cabinet was gathering (all were in Germantown except Hamilton at Trenton and Pickering in the city), trade was fast returning to normal. The weather was cool, bright, windy; the whole town was beautifully clean and neat. Young Tom Adams likewise told his parents that the city was no longer dangerous, news which the Vice-President, always fearful of his health, weighed carefully, for he would have to go there when Congress met.

Young Tom told Mr. Adams that Congress really ought not

to meet in Philadelphia, that Washington ought to prorogue them till a later time. But the Vice-President knew well enough no constitutional power existed to do so. And he also knew that a delayed session would give aid and comfort to the "French Madness" stirred up again by Citizen Genêt. He would have to go to Philadelphia. Mrs. Adams need not go, however. There was no reason for her to endanger herself.

Abigail Adams thought the same. She resolved to stay at Quincy, and invited Tom to come home and spend the winter with her. Tom declined. "If I felt the same degree of alarm that appears to have taken hold of the People at a distance from Philadelphia," he wrote, he would accept. But he believed the city now safe. Mr. Ingersoll, with whom he was studying, had returned, and demanded young Adams come also. Dr. Rush said there was no danger. Law business would be lucrative. Tom returned.

It was surprising, he wrote, after he went back, how quickly a person got over his initial fears, his "impressions of terror," on first entering the city. Tom took lodgings with Mr. Stall in the room left vacant by Johnny Stall's death. "The idea of danger is dissipated in a moment when we perceive thousands walking in perfect security about their customary business, & no ill consequences ensuing from it," he comforted his mother. "Many of the inhabitants are in mourning, which still reminds us of the occasion, but a short time will render it familiar. No person that has [not] been exiled from their usual residence upon such an occasion can realize the joy that is universally felt at meeting a former friend or acquaintance. . . ."

Tom changed his mind about Congress. There was no danger, he thought; and members would realize it once they arrived. General Washington was not so sure. He determined to inspect Lancaster and Reading in person, to see if they could really receive the government. And before he left, he resolved to have a look at Philadelphia. All alone, on the morning of Sunday, November 10, the President rode into the city. Up and down the clean, still streets General Washington rode, looking at everything, bowing slightly to the people he passed, testing the air. He was favorably impressed. All seemed orderly and fresh to him. Congress would not have to move, and they would recognize their safety soon enough. Washington rode back to Germantown, horrified his staff with the news of where he had been, started on his western trip.

Even the arrival of congressmen did not reassure all citizens, however. Some still wrote of the gloom that spread over everything, the appalling memories that made the revival of gaieties in the city a mockery. Susan Dillwyn found the Assembly, the federal government, the great horde of French and other foreigners but a thin cover for emptiness of spirit and exhaustion of the soul. On November 30 John Adams, having reached the city, was still preoccupied with the fever. He wrote Abigail that a deep snow had finally come and would surely extinguish the last traces of disease. But Mr. Jefferson even in December did not know yet which houses were safe to enter.

So the fear hung on. But November was a time of recovery— of moral, psychological, intellectual reconstruction. It was also a time of struggle, for the plague left a thousand loose ends to tie up. The Library Board met, and canceled fines members had incurred during the plague. Father Keating, the only Catholic priest remaining, resumed the care of souls. Some of the Presbyterian ministers came back. The African Society met to find out how much money it had spent. The Pennsylvania Hospital Board came together to formulate a public explanation of their conduct in closing the hospital and suspending meetings. French political riots occurred; one Santo Domingan leader was hurled into the river and nearly drowned before Clarkson could get the city constables there to restore order. People found jobs, starvation was over, wages were high, businessmen resumed all the projects that plague had interrupted. On the streets citizens whom rumor had pronounced dead were seen walking about with the high color and full health of fugitives.

The Committee, in spite of recovery, had still to meet every day. They had to wind up the plague. Israel, Connelly, and Lownes waited on William Hamilton as soon as that gentleman came into town, to discuss compensation for Bush Hill. Hamilton was far from cordial at finding his house turned into a hospital, but he promised not to put the Committee to any inconvenience, or do anything to discommode or injure the more than a hundred patients still at the lazaretto. The managers, meanwhile, began attending Bush Hill only twice a week.

The Guardians of the Poor were reconstituted, and given back their proper tasks. They even agreed to pay poor James Wilson's expenses. On November 12 the Committee threatened to report anyone refusing to clean his house to the grand jury. On the fourteenth they finally announced that applications for admission to Bush Hill had ceased, and proclaimed that their "fugitive brethren" might return.

Dr. Benjamin Duffield, for his services at the hospital, was voted $500. Dr. Devèze, with a memorial of the highest praise, received $1,500. Bush Hill was constituted a permanent hospital for infectious diseases, on the recommendation of Stephen Girard. It was rented for $2,000 for the next year and a half. A careful inventory was taken of everything there—all the beds from the Prison, all the blankets and linens from the Almshouse, all the property of deceased patients, all the firewood, furniture, and food, all the medicines, every bottle of extract of Saturn, Spanish flies, gum alba, ipecacuanha, glauber salts, all the myriad other pharmaceuticals. Then the whole place was leased to the French minister to care for a new boatload of sick and wounded just come in from Santo Domingo.

The orphans still on the Committee's hands—ninety-three in all, thirty-eight of them sucking infants—were given into the care of the General Assembly, whose members, the Committee declared with unintended wit, were "the fathers of the people."

The cargo of vinegar, candles, and lemon juice from Boston was sold—it brought $1,751.87. Joseph Ogden, sexton of Potter's Field, had buried 1,008 paupers; the Committee agreed to pay him five shillings each.

In all these chores there was no interest. The plague was over. Philadelphia was resuming normal life, and wanted to forget the days of pestilence as soon as possible. Even the heroism of the Committee was an uninteresting matter, now that the need for heroism was gone. Gratitude does not belong to cities. The Committee had spent altogether $37,647.19. They had received from all donations $34,402.07. They finished their work with a deficit of $3,245.12. They wanted to make a gift to Mary Saville, the matron of Bush Hill, but they had no funds—not even a few dollars which would have compensated that excellent female for her courageous service.

Many months later, the Committee called a public meeting of all citizens to end their business. A few turned up. Chief Justice Thomas McKean presided. Resolutions of thanks were passed, but nothing else. There the matter rested. Mrs. Saville was never paid, and deficits remained the personal loss of the members of the Committee. John Letchworth, maker of windsor chairs, was out of pocket £1/0/9; what Stephen Girard's losses were, no one could guess.

IV

The whole sore visitation, Ebenezer Hazard wrote, was a lesson. It ought to check the "prevailing taste for enlarging Philadelphia, and crowding so many human beings together on so small a part of earth." He hoped all America would take the hint, and reject the "fashions of the Old World in building great cities."

Governor Mifflin was somewhat more realistic. He had no jurisdiction over the size of cities. All he wanted was to make sure it would not happen again. He placed the militia at Mayor Clarkson's disposal (on November 8, far too late to do any good); he enforced the quarantine law. He did the sober, dull things custom decreed, he eloquently proclaimed a day of general humiliation, thanksgiving, and prayer. And unwittingly, he precipitated a new Rushite controversy.

Anticipating the reassembly of the legislature, Mifflin asked

Mayor Clarkson and the Committee for a complete account of the disaster. The Committee responded with a long description. The Governor also asked the College of Physicians for an account of the cause of the pestilence. At once the old argument sprang to life. Dr. Redman was too feeble to keep the peace. And those who contended for foreign origin had the backing of all the businessmen of the city. The College memorialized the Governor that "No instance has ever occurred of the disease called yellow fever, having originated in this city, or in any other parts of the United States," but that there were frequent instances of its having been imported.

Dr. Rush was appalled at this last bland achievement of the "conspiracy" against him. There was no sense in fighting any longer. On November 5 Rush sent his resignation to the College of Physicians. Though he had helped establish the institution, had been one of its principal ornaments, had applauded its attempts to achieve uniformity in the practice of physic, he would neither compromise his beliefs to accord with the opinions of his colleagues, nor silently acquiesce in a judgment he regarded as mad. He had not caused the split in Philadelphia's great medical community, he insisted; but there was no enduring the treatment he had received. If there must be a split, it would have to be permanent.

Rush could not resist a final gesture. Along with his resignation, with serene pertinence, he sent the College a copy of Sydenham's works.

Ironically enough, his resignation had to be addressed to Dr. Redman as president, sent to Dr. Griffitts as secretary, noted by the treasurer, Benjamin Say. These three officers were almost the only members of the College with whom Rush had no quarrel. Griffitts, back in town, wrote his friend that he was "mortified by the resignation business." "Oh, my friend, search & see if our Resentments are to make us quit places where we can be eminently useful," he pleaded.

But Rush was determined now on his own course. He was compiling his notes, he would write his book, defend his cure.

He would leave Philadelphia if necessary. Frail though he was, he made plans for the future. Fisher took him out for a drive up to Rose Hill, where his son Ben was staying with the Bradfords. The Doctor was too weak to dismount from his carriage, but emaciated and trembling he breathed the fresh country air, and looked upon his son with loving, almost unbelieving eyes. He rode back to Third and Walnut refreshed in flesh and spirit.

And Julia was coming home. She wrote him of her plans. Rush said it was too soon, wait a while. Julia refused to; she packed up, and set a day for her departure. Rush was not sorry. And as the time drew near for a reunion with his wife, he was consumed with impatience. Lonely, isolated from his colleagues, exhausted emotionally and physically, he lived only for the day of their meeting.

I have the deepest sense of your fervent, and unabated affection for me [he wrote Julia], and in the midst of my dangers and distresses, at all times derived consolation from reflecting, that I lived every moment in your remembrance, and was constantly carried by you to the throne of heaven for my preservation. I derived comfort in the near prospects of death likewise, from reflecting upon your extraordinary prudence, your good sense, and pious dispositions, all of which qualified you in an eminent degree to educate our children in a proper manner in case I had been taken from you. This idea, connected with an unshaken faith in God's promises to widows and fatherless children, sometimes suspended for a while my ardent and natural attachment to you and the children, and made me at times willing to part with you provided my death would have advanced the great objects to which I had directed myself.

Each day as he grew stronger he planned to ride to Princeton, or Trenton, or at least Rose Hill to meet her. Would she provide him with a separate bed and room, he asked? For he was still a carrier of infection. And would she "consent to receive me without the usual modes of salutation among long absent, and affectionate friends?"

But each day came new demands upon him; finally his tour of duty at the Pennsylvania Hospital began. He gave up Princeton; then Trenton. He continued to write every morning and night. He praised Julia's "proper and dignified behaviour" during his trials. "I have often said, that you were an uncommon woman," he wrote on November 7.

I can now truly say that you are a GREAT woman, and it will always be my consolation and pleasure (for we should have *pride* in nothing) that in all the letters I have received from my wife and three of my children, not one of them contained a single request, or even hint to me to leave the city, during the late fatal epidemic. For such a wife, and such children, I desire to be thankful.

On the eleventh, Rush began the day by reading the Thirty-seventh Psalm: *Fret not thyself because of evildoers, neither be thou envious against the workers of iniquity.* He was rebuked, he wrote, and humbled by the text. But it was just what Julia had told him about his quarrels with his brethren. The experience was a proper preparation, for next day he learned that she had reached Rose Hill.

My Dearest Julia [he wrote], I want words to describe my emotions upon hearing that the dearest person to me upon the face of the earth is at last within three miles of me, after a long and most distressing separation. A longer and colder ride into the country than usual this morning, has so far exhausted my strength that I fear I could not bear a ride to Rosehill, and afterwards—a first interview with you. I have moreover a patient ill with a disorder which cannot bear the loss of two visits a day at a *certain* hour without the risk of his life. For these reasons I have prevailed upon Mr. Fisher to convey you this letter, with a request to come into town with him, or with an assurance that I will come out (if as well as usual) in the forenoon, and spend the day with you tomorrow.

If you come to town you shall have the front room (now the purest in the house) to yourself. I will sleep in the room adjoining you with the door open between us. Kiss Ben. But—ah—who will kiss, my dear Julia, her

most affectionate husband
BENJAMIN RUSH?

Afterwards

*The evils of pestilence by which this city has lately
been afflicted will probably form an era in its
history.*—CHARLES BROCKDEN BROWN

TRAGEDY does not exist in history, not pure tragedy that sweeps
away the hopes and dreams of men and makes an end to everything; for history is motion, and motion does not stop. The
days of wrath passed by in Philadelphia, life went on, survivors
looked ahead, not back. What men could, they forgot; and what
they could not forget, they translated into usable experience.
But for many years, over all that people did, hung a pall of
apprehension, the gloomy knowledge that plague was now a
dimension of American life, that even Europe's long record of
pestilence could show no greater terror than had stalked abroad
in Philadelphia in 1793.

Some there were who tried to ignore the horrid facts. Charles
Biddle wrote that all the thousands who had died were only
foreigners, interlopers, strangers; that no more than eighty
citizens had perished, and most of these were foreign-born.
Such capricious error may have comforted Charles Biddle, but
no one else believed it. Too many homes had been touched,
too many families broken. More honest was Mathew Carey, as
he told the frightful legion of the dead.

Even before the disease had gone, Carey had his history set
up in his printing shop, ready for sale. It appeared on November
14: *A Short Account of the Malignant Fever, Lately Prevalent
in Philadelphia: with a Statement of the Proceedings That Took
Place on the Subject in Different Parts of the United States.*
Everyone wanted a copy; a second edition came in nine days,

280

a third the next week (November 30). The third was "improved" by the addition of a *List of the Names of the Persons Buried in the Several Graveyards of the City and Liberties of Philadelphia from August 1st, to November 9th, 1793*—the necrology that people demanded.

Carey kept his type standing, ran off further printings, added new data in his page forms. As edition succeeded edition, he gradually fashioned an extraordinary book, a substantial souvenir of disaster written with clarity and spirit, with lively awareness of the human values of the plague and a canny appraisal of the market. The *Short Account* grew into a long relation, and into a highly successful investment. A fourth edition came at the end of the year, adding names of the dead from November 9 through the middle of December; an "improved" fourth edition in two issues the next month (January 16) contained appendices describing plagues in London and Marseilles. Four editions in French translation followed one another; a certain Carl Erdmann did a German version which Samuel Saur in Chestnut Hill and J. Bailey at Lancaster both printed "für den Verfasser"; London reprints appeared, and in Haarlem a translation in Dutch.

Abroad, it was the narrative which sold Carey's book, but at home it was the necrology, those endless lists of people who had died. Rush might claim great cures—"to tell you of all the people who have been bled and purged out of the grave in our city, would require a book nearly as large as the Philadelphia directory," he wrote. And rumor might be confounded by the living presence of persons reported dead; but Carey's lists contained the indisputable truth of this calamity. He counted 4,044, counted and named them. Yet even this was not the whole, for nearly everyone could mention others who were not named in Carey's book. Dolly Todd's little child, for example, and Sebastian Ale, and many more Carey did not list.

Nor did numbers alone tell the story. Ten of the doctors, ten of the ministers, even more merchants, even more lawyers, these of the city's great were among the dead. And hundreds upon hundreds who were merely names, and countless nameless children; laborers, servants, artisans of all trades, Negroes known only by a nickname—Carey's list was a cross section of Philadelphia. The total number of deaths cannot be computed; it will never be known. Carey's figures show half the houses closed, half the inhabitants fled; probably more than five thousand perished in the city alone.

But it was not the fact of death that people dreaded; death was familiar to them all. Every year, without a plague, a quarter of all children born died before they learned to walk; half of all mankind perished before the age of nine. What shocked people was a sudden mass of death, the uneasy fear that would forever after go with living in a city. Some left Philadelphia, never to return. Others provided themselves with summer homes whither they could retreat in the feverish season. Still others began to work for the improvement of the city itself, and for the expansion of medical science.

At once, of course, the doctors assembled their notes into lectures. Rush opened his class at the University with "a performance of deep and touching interest," Charles Caldwell wrote, "never, I think, to be forgotten (while his memory endures) by any one who listened to it." And Griffitts lectured on the plague and Barton, and others, even Kuhn. The medical literature of yellow fever was beginning. It grew every year, as the fever returned.

For return the fever did, in 1794, and 1796, and 1797, and 1798, and for many years thereafter. Seven great plagues and many lesser visitations came to the city in the course of a generation, and as the nineteenth century wore on yellow fever spread to countless American towns and states, to Baltimore, Mobile, New Orleans, to most of the settled parts of the land south and west. All the scenes of horror, all the desperation, all the controversies and doubts of the months through which Philadelphia had just passed, were repeated again and again. The city itself kept its quarantine, its hospital, its orphan asylum; it developed ways of coping with the plague. In 1798 huge encampments of tents in the open fields by the Schuylkill and in the Northern Liberties were pitched for the poor from squalid districts, quite as Dr. Currie had recommended. Congress passed a law giving the President power to call it together elsewhere than its regular place whenever pestilence or other hazard to life and health existed; the Pennsylvania Assembly vested special authority in the Governor. Bequests to the city corporation for relief of fever victims became a familiar charity (one of them, John Bleakley's fund, is still being administered); and, overwhelmed by repeated calamities, Philadelphia erected its great public waterworks, in hope of cleansing the city of its fetid miasmas.

Book after book came from the doctors—from Rush and Currie, Devèze, Nassy, Isaac Cathrall, the College of Physicians, from all who could find a publisher. The yellow fever, before the death of the young men whose first plague was 1793, became the most thoroughly written-about disease in medicine.

We have forgotten this huge literature today, because we live after Walter Reed; but until 1902 every visitation of the black vomit had a special importance, and Philadelphia's great plague, the first of a long series, attracted all the writers of medical history. It attracted other writers, too, those who saw moral and humanistic values in the plague. The Reverend Henry Helmuth put his sober reflections into a book; so did Samuel Stearns, J.U.D., and many more. Elegiac odes in hideous metre seemed always to have an audience. Philadelphia businessmen apprehensive lest the trade of the city decline, lawyers, travelers, diarists, and compilers of city directories all wrote of the plague in attempts to explain it away. Noah Webster regarded yellow fever as a national problem, to be solved on a national scale; he published essays and two books on the subject. Greatest of all literary monuments to the plague of 1793 was Charles Brockden Brown's career, for three of his novels, *The Man at Home, Arthur Mervyn,* and *Ormond,* described the fever in Philadelphia with all the somber passion and turgid prose of which he was so abundantly capable. ("I want no succor; vex

me not with your entreaties and offers"; cries a sufferer in
Arthur Mervyn. "Fly from this spot; linger not a moment, lest
you participate my destiny and rush upon your death.") Brown
as a misanthropic young Quaker of twenty-three had actually
seen the early days of the fever in the city before he fled to New
York in September. His books have frequently been used as
historical evidence; they are scarcely that, but they are the first
literary accounts of the plague in all its mysterious majesty,
all its grim and fantastic senselessness.

They are the first of several such accounts, for this plague
has appeared in various guises in American letters. It was the
theme of a novel in 1943 (*Judith,* by Janet Whitney); S. Weir
Mitchell devoted stirring chapters to it in *The Red City* (1907);
and Longfellow's Evangeline finally discovered her Gabriel in
Philadelphia in the midst of the pestilence as

. . . on a Sabbath morn, through the streets, deserted and silent,
Wending her quiet way, she entered the door of the almshouse.

Now curiously, all this literature distorted rather than illumi-
nated the truth about the disaster of 1793. Myths, legends,
folklore passed from one writer to another, accepted and believed; details of 1798 were mixed and commingled with those
of 1793, even the facts as given by Carey and Rush (the most
available sources) were ignored or warped out of shape. Just
as Longfellow should have known from reading Carey that the
Almshouse was the last place a fever victim would have been
found, so Weir Mitchell should have realized that Dr. Rush
was no simple combination of piety and malice, easily explained;
and LaRoche, in his huge work on yellow fever, should have
read what was there to see rather than search for hints to support his prejudices.

But men do not learn from history; and the sentiments customary among historians rarely permit them to indulge in
austere observation. It was tradition, not truth, which grew into
literature, tradition American and optimistic. So irresistible
were the currents of nationalistic thought that the great French

doctors, the Santo Domingan volunteers, the failure of Americans and the successes of the refugees at Bush Hill, were all but forgotten. LaRoche paid tribute to Devèze, but it was Rush, Griffitts, Physick, and Caldwell who entered into the tradition of medical and popular writing, who became the celebrated figures of the plague. Of all the opponents of mercury and bleeding, only Girard was held in memory, and this for his heroism rather than for his theory.

Facts do not make tradition; they are swept away as it forms. But tradition makes history in its own terms, and gives each disaster such place in knowledge as men can know and use. This process begins as soon as disaster is over, as soon as those who survive begin to forget a part of their experience, and devote the unforgettable remnant to some use. Afterwards, disaster is tortured by reason, tragedy averted by the simple persistence of living.

After the plague of 1793, the widow of Andrew Adgate began to take in boarders. Afterwards, both Quaker and Catholic leadership were rebuilt. Afterwards, Peter Helm quietly returned to his coopering shop, to come forth again in every civic crisis for many years as a man skilled in goodness; while Stephen Girard resumed his lonely existence, going from one service to another, rising higher in the esteem of Philadelphians, withdrawing further from their midst, finally crowning his endless efforts with the largest bequest to public charities that the modern world had ever seen.

Afterwards, Dr. Leib and Israel Israel squandered their gifts in local partisanship. James Mease, cursed with a bountiful inheritance, fiddled away his time in hobbies. Physick and Cathrall achieved medical eminence in this country, Devèze abroad. Young Coxe and Barton and Woodhouse pursued scientific careers with great distinction, Charles Caldwell in the same pursuit revealed himself a fool. Benjamin Say passed on his modest gifts to his far greater son, the father of American entomology.

Afterwards, individuals reassembled their strengths, formed

new patterns of life and of fellowship. The great truth of the fever had been the decay and rebirth of the whole city as men shared the realities of every day. Individuals did not shape, but were shaped by, the sudden occasion they had not created, the inexorable movement they could not stay, the inevitable recovery they did not themselves achieve.

Life went on in Philadelphia; but no one who lived through the Yellow Fever of 1793 was ever quite the same again.

Notes

ALL footnotes have been cut out of this book, under the impression that they annoy more readers than they help. But I want to make clear that this is an account from the sources, not a piece of imagination or fiction. When an historian says his work is true, he means a rather special thing; for what he has actually performed is a sort of reconstruction, a re-creation. His facts, his sources, are accessible to anyone; his use of them is his own particular contribution to understanding, and to morality. Now every fact in this book, every opinion attributed to a contemporary, even the occasional conversations recorded, are all in the sources. I have invented none of them. These notes are inserted to satisfy the curiosity of such as may wonder, that so much can be known, of even the simple, unpretentious part of society, so many years ago.

The Sources. The plague left an abundant record. In general, my most important sources were:

(1) The Papers of Dr. Benjamin Rush in the Library Company of Philadelphia, including great numbers of letters from and addressed to him, various manuscript writings on fever, and such items as the Mitchell manuscript responsible for Rush's Ten-and-Ten inspiration, his letters to Hodge and Wistar, the dying letter of Johnny Stall to his father, and so on.

(2) The volume privately published by Alexander Biddle in 1892, called *Old Family Letters Relating to the Yellow Fever.* This consists of letters written by Dr. Rush to his wife between August 21 and November 12, 1793, those incomparable letters, badly edited by Mr. Biddle, but restored to sense and meaning by notes Lyman H. Butterfield has most kindly added to the Free Library's copy. These notes Mr. Butterfield made from the original letters, now in the possession of Josiah C. Trent, M.D., of Durham, North Carolina, through whose permission they were used.

(3) The *Federal Gazette* published daily by Andrew Brown all during the fever. I used the copy belonging to the Library Company of Philadelphia.

(4) The little books, descriptions, or tracts written on the plague by those who lived through it. Dr. William Pepper presented a very large collection of these books to the Free Library of Philadelphia,

and this collection was what first aroused my interest in the subject. Subsequently other books not in the Pepper collection were consulted at the College of Physicians of Philadelphia, the Library Company, the Historical Society of Pennsylvania, and the American Philosophical Society. To list all these books by title would be of slight value. Those by Carey, Rush, Currie, Nassy, Devèze, Noah Webster, and Cathrall, and one anonymous *Account* (probably written by James Hardie), proved the most useful; the books of the Negroes Jones and Allen and of Parson Helmuth likewise furnished information not available elsewhere. Many of these books on the fever are listed in Evans' *American Bibliography*.

(5) The Minutes of the Committee, the original manuscript of which in Caleb Lownes' hand is in the Library Company of Philadelphia, and which was printed by order of the City Council in the year 1848.

(6) Stephen Girard's Papers in Girard College were made available to me by the board of that institution; and I placed much reliance upon MacMaster's *Life* of Girard, a thorough study of the original papers.

In addition to these major sources, a good many minor sources have been consulted. There were many of them; I could have gone on reading sources indefinitely, for every collection of American manuscripts in the country probably has something on this plague. I drew an arbitrary line. Washington, Jefferson, and Hamilton I investigated only through standard published editions of writings or letters. Thomas Adams' letters to his father and mother are in the Adams Family Papers and were copied for me by Henry Adams, Esq.

Some Ebenezer Hazard letters are published in the Massachusetts Historical Society Collections. In the Connecticut Historical Society are the Oliver Wolcott Manuscripts, including letters from Dawson and other Treasury clerks used in this volume.

At the Historical Society of Pennsylvania are Hazard Family Papers; the Maria Dickinson Logan Papers with letters of Mary Norris of Chester and Deborah Norris Logan, Dr. George Logan's wife; the Wallace Papers with letters of Judge William Bradford; a long Benjamin Smith Barton letter on the fever; Stephen Girard's Bush Hill Hospital Accounts; letters of the merchant John Welsh; and scattered letters and other manuscripts in the various great autograph collections of the Society.

The Library Company of Philadelphia, in addition to the Rush Papers and the printed books collection, also has manuscript diaries and letters of the plague year, among them the vivid letters of Susanna Dillwyn to her father in London. The Minute Books of the Library Company directors, like the records of other institutions, take ample notice of the fever.

The College of Physicians of Philadelphia, in addition to its printed books, has manuscript accounts of the plague by John Redman Coxe and J. Pemberton, lectures by some of the doctors, and students' notes.

Other manuscript sources were used more or less at random. Two letters of Samuel Wetherill were shown me by a descendant; Dr. Noel J. Cortes, Dr. John Munroe, and Mr. Irving Morris all supplied me with Thomas Rodney letters. Mr. Joseph S. Miller studied Andrew Adgate letters in his possession at my request. Sale catalogues of autograph dealers (collected since 1891 by the Free Library) supplied some letters and many leads.

William Matthews' bibliography of American diaries before 1861 was most helpful as I checked the published materials. Charles Caldwell's autobiography, and diaries or autobiographies of Jacob Hiltzheimer, Samuel Breck, Elizabeth Drinker, and Charles Biddle, were among my most important sources, though the plague is at least mentioned in almost all other diaries that covered this year in the eastern states.

Dr. Redman's lecture before the College on September 7, 1793, was not printed until 1865. Frequently, original material appears in the text of later books, such as Dr. Bond's lecture of 1766, which is printed in Norris' *The Early History of Medicine in Philadelphia* (1886) ; or Dr. Clark's letter describing fever in Dominica in July 1793, published in a volume of *Facts and Observations* by the College of Physicians in 1798.

The *Journal of the Senate* records the details of the brief legislative session in September; the *Executive Minutes* of Governor Thomas Mifflin (a volume in Pennsylvania Archives, ninth series) contain what little the Governor did from his pleasant retreat at Falls of Schuylkill.

Hardie's *Philadelphia Directory* of 1793 and his second directory the following year were indispensable in identifying people. Benjamin Davies' *Some Account of the City of Philadelphia* (1794) is an excellent description of the community, its social and economic structure.

General and special works in medical history I have, of course, used extensively. Packard and Shryock are invaluable in setting the point of view, Flexner's *Doctors on Horseback* brilliantly describes the drama of the plague. Many articles in the periodical *Annals of Medical History* furnished both data and interpretive suggestions. General works in Philadelphia history are both numerous and confused (probably none of the older American cities has had its history so badly written as this one), but contain a great deal of obscure information, and much of the information in this book is certainly obscure.

Nathan G. Goodman's biography, *Benjamin Rush*, Charles Coleman Sellers' *Charles Willson Peale*, J. Bennett Nolan's *Printer Strahan's Account Book*, Charles F. Jenkins' studies of Washington and Jefferson in Germantown, Charles Wesley's life of Richard Allen, and all other apposite biographies have been consulted.

Finally, historical curiosity, institutional pride, and genealogical study in the nineteenth century produced many pamphlets which preserved data otherwise surely lost. Reports of yellow fever committees, of water boards, necrological notices of eminent characters (such as Philip Syng Physick, Andrew Brown, or Dr. James Gardette), church celebrations (Absalom Jones's St. Thomas Church held several), biographical orations and addresses, and so on, all add details to the whole; in 1854 was printed such a pamphlet, *Abstract of Title to the Bush Hill Estate* . . .

The Title. "Bring Out Your Dead!" is the cry tradition assigns to the carters in the great plague in London, 1664/5, and to this visitation as well. In both cases it is only tradition; probably the picture of continual repetition of this doleful cry is but a romantic invention. In London it is hard to prove from the sources, and in Philadelphia no contemporary even mentions these words. The impression one gets is of carters' entering houses and with their own hands carrying the dead out to their wagons. James M. Beck attributed this cry to our plague; but Beck's gift for irresponsible invention in history was uncommon. Yet several Philadelphia families preserve a tradition of the fever in which this cry is used, and some have written me of stories their grandmothers heard from *their* grandmothers, in which "Bring Out Your Dead!" occurs.

Weather and Climate. It is curiously true that every day's weather during this period is perfectly recorded in the sources. The astronomer David Rittenhouse wrote down barometer and thermometer readings, and wind and weather conditions, every morning at six and every afternoon at three. Thus, when I say the wind was in Rush's face as he walked up Second Street, I learn it from Rittenhouse's note that the wind that day was north; and his temperature readings prove that August 19 was "cloudy, a little cooler than usual lately." All the writers on the fever discussed the climate and its changes, newspapers described the erratic behavior of nature, Noah Webster particularly collected signs of sinister forces at work in air, sea, and sky. The foul smells in the city were carefully traced to their source by contagionists.

Location of the plague scene in present-day Philadelphia. Some of the buildings mentioned can still be seen in Philadelphia, among them the State House group (Independence Hall and City Hall), St. George's Church, the American Philosophical Society, the Pennsylvania Hospital, and "Smith's Folly" out in Germantown. Water Street, Elfreth's Alley, Newmarket Street, Queen Street, and a few other survivals of eighteenth-century blocks preserve the spirit of an older time, and help one understand how any disease might flourish in the "Red City."

Where Ricketts' circus was in 1793, today the P.S.F.S. sky-scraper stands. Where the Loganian library became the orphan house, today the Saturday Evening Post is published. The grounds of the Walnut Street Prison today are occupied by the Penn Mutual Insurance Company and other buildings.

Bush Hill mansion was located on the site of the present United States Mint, and the farm included Old Central High School, the Cathedral of SS. Peter and Paul, the Municipal Court, Eastern State Penitentiary, and a good deal beside.

In surrounding regions one can see many houses that were standing while the fever raged, and Major Piercy's tombstone still rises by a country road in Jersey.

The cannon. Janet Whitney, James M. Beck, and many other writers have preserved the legend of a large cannon booming through the city every day. But the sources are completely silent about a cannon, except for the one day when Hiltzheimer describes the Artillery Company actually dragging it about—one day only. Even then, it was only a little cannon. It would make a smart report, but it would not boom. I think it was used only this once, and that the phrase, "flash gunpowder and other salutary preparations through the streets," meant simple burning. Captain Thornton's complaints to the Governor mention only "duty in the city," by which he probably meant Fort Mifflin; they do not mention street patrols. Unquestionably, one day of the annoying cannon was enough.

This Plague and Later Plagues. Each time the fever returned, new horrors occurred, new stories were told. I find that many people who have read or heard part of this book expect their favorite stories of later plagues to appear in it. To later plagues belong William Cobbett and his great feud with Rush, the tent cities along the Schuylkill bank, the licentiousness and depravity of the city, and many of the anecdotes of Dr. Rush. Of all the visitations of the fever, this one in 1793, first of the series, and that of 1798, were the worst.

The Doctors and Their Medicines. Medical history is usually written in terms of the great men, as if what the leaders in medical thought and invention did gained immediate general acceptance. Of course this is not true, for there are always the great mass of doctors who lag behind the leaders. The actual practice of medicine has its history, too, though it is very difficult to get at.

Empirics are easier to find than proper doctors. They advertised in newspapers, Dr. Rush wrote about them, Dr. Say published a life of his colorful father, Hardie's *Directory* lists many of these curious people. They deserve more study, these dentists and aurists, cancer doctors, quacks, and charlatans, by medical as well as social historians.

I have a list of more than eighty respectable doctors in the city, more than a hundred in the city and county, compiled from newspapers, directories, and all other sources. Obviously, when Rush said only three doctors were on their feet, he didn't mean three out of all these. Now if this kind of list were made for all American cities from 1760 to 1800 (a comparatively simple task), it would teach us a great deal about medicine in the Revolutionary period which we do not know. The number of Rush's former students practicing could then be put in its proper relationship with the total number of doctors practicing, and other quantitative studies might be made.

A study of the wonderful medicines the doctors used would better be done by a poet than a scientist (who would be offended) or an historian (who would miss all the beauty of the task). John Redman Coxe described these medicines a little later on, when he edited the *American Dispensatory* (1808) and compiled a medical dictionary. Some of the strangest words—"lenitive chologoque," for example—are still used, and would be understood at once by your corner druggist; but "inquiline humors," "excrementitious fluids," and similar phrases are now considered a bit old-fashioned.

Venesection. Clearly, there is a puzzle to be solved in connection with Rush's bloodletting, particularly to explain how so many patients recovered from this depleting regimen. One possibility is that the amount of blood actually drawn was unwittingly exaggerated; but against this are the specific counts by ounces in the cases of Drs. Mease, Griffitts, and Physick. Dr. O. H. Perry Pepper, in *Transactions and Studies of the College of Physicians,* 4th Ser., Vol. 14, No. 3., Dec. 1946, pp. 121-26, discusses the issue, but does not reach an explanation. The puzzle is that so many can be proved to have recovered (although of course great numbers did not). I cannot solve this puzzle.

Statistical Records of the Plague. This fever occurred before any systematic use of statistics was in vogue. It is therefore hard to know just what the figures were. Carey used the lists of burial grounds, but many fugitives died outside the city, and numbers within were doubtless buried without registration. His tables are misleading in another respect, for he shows only three persons buried in the Jewish cemetery, only two in the Universalist. Now the latter may be correct, but the former certainly does not indicate the whole number of Jewish deaths; several others can be named from other sources. The statistics gathered by the Committee, showing the numbers of houses closed, inhabitants fled and of those remaining, the dead, come closer to a picture of the operation of the fever in the city. Hardest of all to describe are the first cases.

John Redman Coxe's manuscript account avers that the earliest attack occurred on July 27, the victim a Kensington dock hand. Other doctors refer to cases in July, but they are vague about them. No understandable figures at all show the number of cases at any one time in September, October, or November; I am not inclined to accept Mr. Jefferson, Colonel Pickering, or Oliver Wolcott as qualified or informed observers.

The Santo Domingans. The refugees have been described in a number of works recently; I am particularly grateful for Frances Sergeant Childs' *French Refugee Life in the United States.* But most of what I said of them came from the Philadelphia newspapers, or from refugee accounts. (Incidentally, Moreau de St. Mery did not reach the city until several months after the plague of 1793 had ended; neither did Prince Talleyrand.) Obviously, the presence of yellow fever victims from the sugar islands, whom *aegypti* could feed on before biting native Philadelphians, was a primary social cause of the epidemic. Ordinary commerce with the islands would have brought some fever victims back; but the enormous number of them in 1793 was unquestionably responsible for the magnitude of the plague.

Caldwell at Bush Hill. Charles Caldwell, in his autobiography, gives the impression that he was at Bush Hill through most of the plague. Actually, he could not have stayed there more than a few days at the most. He went after the establishment; he was gone before Girard and Helm arrived. His experience was really very limited, even more limited than the four American doctors who occasionally visited Bush Hill before September 16. But typically, he made it seem enormous. Caldwell remained a Rushite in bleeding and purging. He probably knew nothing of Devèze's remedy.

The Unethanneh Toqef. Of course, Mikveh Israel was, and still is, a Sephardic-rite congregation, and I am uneasy about using an Ashkenazic prayer in writing of their Rosh Hashanah celebration. The large majority of Philadelphia's Jews, however, was not of unmixed Spanish-Portuguese descent; most of them knew the German tradition, and I have no doubt that the *Unethanneh Toqef* was familiar to them all.

The Carey Controversy. Carey's unfortunate slur on the Negro nurses in his first edition provoked Jones and Allen to write their book in rejoinder. In addition, "Argus" published an attack on Carey, alleging that he had fled the city the day he was put on the Committee, that the cold reception he endured in the country drove him back, that he would not relieve the poor or be seen with vagabonds. Carey answered this in an *Address of Mathew Carey to the Public,* a copy of which I saw through the kindness of Miss Mabel Zahn. The publisher confesses that he left the city on September 16, but affirms that he had told the Committee of his departure in advance. Dr. Currie was sitting next to him, he declares, and can vouch for his statement. He traveled through Virginia and Maryland settling accounts, returned as soon as he could, and worked hard and loyally at his Committee tasks. The charge that he made money from his pamphlet he refutes, and points out that Clarkson and Lownes asked him to write the history of the plague. Clearly, Mathew Carey was both innocent and irreproachable in his conduct. He explained his unfortunate sentence about the Negroes in a way which the candid reader must regard as satisfactory.

Index

(Physicians in America during the yellow fever, mentioned in this book, are indicated by the word "Dr.")